Testosterone:
A Man's Guide

*Practical Tips for Boosting Sexual,
Physical, and Mental Vitality*

Nelson Vergel, BsChE, MBA
Co-Author of "Built To Survive"

Disclaimer

The information contained in this publication is for educational purposes only, and is in no way a substitute for the advice of a qualified health care provider. Appropriate medical therapy and the use of pharmaceutical compounds like testosterone should be tailored for the individual, as no two individuals are alike. The author does not recommend self-medicating with any compound, as you should consult with a qualified medical doctor who can determine your individual situation. Any use of the information presented in this publication for personal medical therapy is done strictly at your own risk and no responsibility is implied or intended on the part of the author, contributors, or the publisher.

Cover Design: Rob Tomlin, Houston, Texas
Vergel, Nelson, 1959
Testosterone: A Man's Guide

Second edition
ISBN 978-0-9837739-1-7
Medicine, Health, Nutrition, Chemistry, Endocrinology
Library of Congress Control Number: 2010933334

Milestones Publishing
P.O. Box 667223
Houston, TX 77266

For updates, visit testosteronewisdom.com, the blog testosteronewisdom. blogspot.com or the Facebook page called "Testosterone Replacement Therapy Discussion".

Reviews

Unlike authors of other testosterone books, Nelson's search for health compelled him to try most of the options that he describes, so he provides practical "how-to" information. Aided by his chemical engineering degree and obsession for scientific data, he adds his own personal experience as he demystifies all testosterone myths by reviewing published studies. He also makes it easy for the reader to find a doctor in their area that prescribes testosterone by providing easily searchable directories. For those with no insurance, he shows you how to apply for patient assistance programs and research studies, and to obtain economical gels from compounding pharmacies (an important source that most men and doctors fail to access). To counteract side effects, he shows specific protocols to treat the enlargement of breasts and shrinkage of testicles that some men experience when using testosterone, and how to prevent potential cardiovascular problems caused by testosterone's increase of red blood cells. Unlike other books that claim that testosterone is the main solution to improve erectile strength, Nelson cautions that extra measures sometimes are needed by some men, and he specifies each one of them. He also adds to-the-point information about nutrition, supplements and exercise to maximize the benefits of testosterone. And he uncovers the false claims surrounding supplements believed to increase testosterone naturally. This book can save a lot of time and trouble for any man that is serious about his health!
—**Dr. Carlos Barrero, Guadalajara, Mexico**

For men, this book is a must read. For men considering testosterone replacement therapy (TRT), this book is required reading! TRT is currently be taken by millions of men and millions more have the diagnosis of hypogonadism that will have a better quality of life on TRT. Men hate going to a doctor and are even more hesitant to discuss or ask questions related to their sexuality. Nelson Vergel's newest book,"Testosterone: A Man's Guide"; is the first and only book that approaches these subjects in a friendly and informative manner for men. This book provides the bare knuckles' how to tips, on the treatment of male hypogonadism. The book states how to maximize benefits while minimizing any side effects. And the book is written by someone with over two decades of personal experience. This makes the book that more valuable. Nelson Vergel's knowledge, experience, skill, and education on the subject of TRT have been proven in his prior writings, including Built to Survive: A Comprehensive Guide to the Medical Use of Anabolic Steroids, Nutrition and Exercise for HIV (+)

men and women. Nelson deeply cares about men's health. It is more than a passing interest. For him, it is a matter of life and living. I am humbled to be a part of the book. Do yourself a favor and be good to yourself. Get the book!
—**Dr. Michael Scally, Houston**

Nelson Vergel, in his new book "Testosterone: A Man's Guide" masterfully educates his readership about testosterone deficiency and what to do about it. I applaud Nelson for tackling a complex topic and providing a nuanced, important and very helpful guide regarding the under recognized syndrome of testosterone deficiency. As a physician who treats testosterone deficient male patients I have found Nelson's book so informatively and clearly written that I have recommended his book to medical colleagues. Importantly, reading this book has further educated me about testosterone. Nelson, points out that testosterone deficiency can cause many problems for men including depression, low energy, irritability, difficulty concentrating, and body shape changes, in addition to loss of interest in sex and impaired sexual prowess. Since most men and even many physicians fail to recognize the meaning of these symptoms, testosterone deficiency is often not diagnosed causing many men needless suffering. Finally, it should be pointed out that this book is not inappropriately enthusiastic about testosterone replacement therapy. But rather it very carefully spells out the need for an accurate diagnosis of testosterone deficiency, an analysis of the potential benefits and drawbacks of treatment, and the importance of the proper monitoring of therapy. I hope Nelson's book gains the wide readership it deserves because of its power to improve the health and quality of life of countless individuals.
—**Dr. Paul Curtis Bellman, New York**

I would like to thank my partner, Timothy Baker, MD, for his support and the many hours that he spent editing this book, and my friend, Rob Tomlin, for his great probono cover design work. And last but not least, thanks to all the patients and physicians in the past 20 years I have met in my lectures and online forums who have shared their health tips so that others could benefit from their search. I hope that I have become a vessel for all that communal wisdom.

You are about to read the latest and most updated information on testosterone as of the time of this book's print. Unlike most books, this one is written by someone like you who was in search of ways to feel and perform better.

As you will soon find out, there is a lot we know about testosterone, but a lot more will emerge as new research study data and products are available. I want to ensure that you stay updated and connected to the community of men around the world who are already taking charge of their health in a progressive way.

To stay on top of the latest in the field, please do not hesitate to visit and subscribe to (one or several, depending on your preference):

Website: TestosteroneWisdom.com

Blog: testosteronewisdom.blogspot.com

Facebook page: Testosterone Replacement Therapy Discussion

Yahoo group:
health.groups.yahoo.com/group/MensHealthAdvances

How to Order More Copies of This Book:
This book is available at Amazon.com and on TestosteroneWisdom.com in print and ebook formats. For orders outside the United States where amazon is not available, mail a bank-check or money order for US$30 (which includes shipping and handling) to: Milestones Publishing. P.O.Box 667223. Houston, TX 77266

A Spanish translation, "La Testosterona: La Mejor Guia Para Hombres," is available on Amazon.com in kindle and print versions.

I welcome comments via my email nelsonvergel@gmail.com and reviews on this book's Amazon page. I reply to all emails, so do not hesitate even if it is to say hello!

ABOUT THE AUTHOR

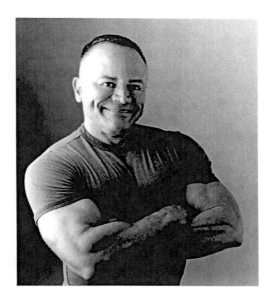

Nelson Vergel is the co-author of the book "Built to Survive: A Comprehensive Guide on the Medical Use of Anabolic Therapies, Nutrition and Exercise for HIV+ Women and Men" and the founder of the Body Positive Wellness Clinic and Program for Wellness Restoration (powerusa.org) in Houston. He holds a bachelor's degree in chemical engineering from McGill University and an MBA from the University of Houston. A tireless patient advocate for over 20 years, his writing is accessible and jam-packed full of practical information. He weaves the latest research data with first-hand experience and useful tips—the result of years of trial and error experience. He strives to help his readers live healthier lives without having to "reinvent the wheel" in their search for solutions.

Nelson discovered the benefits of testosterone replacement therapy in 1993 after doing his own research to reverse his life threatening spiral with fatigue and wasting syndrome. Testosterone allowed him to regain his health and energy as he built lean body mass needed for his survival. This in turn bought him time to survive HIV until effective therapies were introduced in 1996. Convinced that testosterone saved him from dying of wasting syndrome, he embarked on a lecture crusade that has helped thousands of people live healthier lives through the medical use of hormones, exercise, nutrition, supplementation, and other wellness-related therapies.

After spending four years as an active member of metabolic disorders research committee at AIDS Clinical Trials Group of the U. S. National Institutes of Health, he became a leading research advocate and has been featured in numerous publications for his expertise and perspective. He has authored and participated in several studies on the use of hormones, exercise and supplementation that have demystified those approaches for clinical applications. He has lectured at over 60 scientific conferences and to over 500 physician and patient groups, is an expert advisor at TheBody.com, and actively manages the largest online health support group for those living with HIV (pozhealth at yahoogroups.com). Because of his dedicated efforts to help others, the Mayor of the City of Houston, Lee Brown, proclaimed September 13, 2001 as "Nelson Vergel Day."

In this book, Nelson wants to share his health wisdom with men around the world, regardless of their health status. It is his hope that no man has to suffer needlessly from a condition that is easily resolved if diagnosed, treated and monitored by a properly trained physician. He believes that an educated patient can help physicians be great partners in the search for health.

ABBREVIATIONS

Androgen Deficiency in the Aging Male	ADAM
benign prostatic hyperplasia	BPH
dehydroepiandrosterone	DHEA
dihydrotestosterone	DHT
digital rectal examination	DRE
Drug Enforcement Agency	DEA
estrogen receptor	ER
follicle-stimulating hormone	FSH
Food and Drug Administration	FDA
gonadotropin-releasing hormone	GnRH
health management organization	HMO
high-density lipoprotein	HDL
highly active antiretroviral therapy	HAART
human chorionic gonadotropin	HCG
human growth hormone	HGH
hypothalamic-pituitary-gonadal axis	HPGA
hypothalamic-pituitary-testicular axis	HPTA
low density lipoprotein	LDL
luteinizing hormone	LH
nitric oxide	NO
over-the-counter	OTC
Physician's Desk Reference	PDR
prostatic specific antigen	PSA
selective androgen receptor modulators	SARMs
sex hormone binding globulin	SHBG
testosterone replacement therapy	TRT

TABLE OF CONTENTS

About the Author   vii

List of Figures   xii

List of Tables   xiii

Chapter 1 Introduction   1

Chapter 2 Testosterone 101   4

History of Testosterone   4

What Is Testosterone and How Does it Work?   4

What Are the Symptoms of Low Testosterone?   9

Determining If You Have Testosterone Deficiency   10

Causes of Testosterone Deficiency   11

Diagnosis of Testosterone Deficiency   13

Chapter 3 Testosterone Replacement Options   19

Top Mistakes in Testosterone Replacement Therapy   19

Testosterone Formulations   23

Chapter 4 Monitoring Testosterone Replacement Therapy   70

Ensuring Prostate Health   73

Ensuring Liver Health   81

Monitoring Blood Pressure   82

Avoiding Enlarged Breast (Gynecomastia)   83

Medications and Products That Can Cause Gynecomastia   84

Keeping Cholesterol (Lipids) in Check   85

Hypothalamic-Pituitary-Gonadal Axis (HPGA) Dysfunction   94

Chapter 5 When Testosterone is Not Enough   98
When Testosterone Replacement Doesn't Lead to Better
Erections and More Energy

Chapter 6 Supplements   115
Supplements That Claim to Improve Sexual Function
and/or Testosterone

Chapter 7 Miscellaneous Health Tips to Support
Healthy Testosterone   120

Chapter 8 Testosterone Replacement, Side Effects
and Management   131
Interview With Dr. Michael Scally

Resources

Appendix A: Medical History Form   149

Appendix B: Resources and Patient Assistance Programs   155

Appendix C: Frequently Asked Questions
about Compounding   160

Appendix D: How to Find Physicians Who Treat
Hypogonadism   164

Appendix E: Directory of Testosterone Studies   166

Index   181

LIST OF FIGURES

1. Hormonal cascade that regulates testosterone production in males 5
2. Testosterone metabolites 7
3. Testosterone fractions in the blood 8
4. Target organs - beneficial and negative effects of testosterone 9
5. Testosterone decreases as we age as SHBG increases 14
6. Variations in testosterone blood levels during the day for young and older men 15
7. Testosterone Enanthate 250 mg Administered IM every 3 Weeks 27
8. Blood testosterone, estradiol and DHT concentration curves after a 200 mg injection of testosterone enanthate every two weeks 28
9. Testosterone injection sites 36
10. Testosterone blood levels are more stable with testosterone gels 39
11. Commercially available testosterone gels in the United States 40
12. Body areas where gels are usually applied 42
13. TopiClick Applicator for a compounded testosterone cream 44
14. Axiron, an underarm testosterone gel 62
15. The prostate and surrounding organs 74
16. Injection of Trimix on the side of the penis 103

LIST OF TABLES

1. Benifits of Normalizing Testosterone   10
2. Laboratory Ranges and Codes   16
3. HCG Dilution Table   52
4. Monitoring Testosterone Therapy:
   What the Consensus Guidelines Say   72
5. Oral Erectile Dysfunction Drugs-
   How long do they stay in the body?   101

-1-

Introduction

My relationship with testosterone replacement has been a long and fruitful one. I was diagnosed with low testosterone in 1993 at the age of 34 after I had been living with HIV for 11 years. I had lost 14 pounds unintentionally, felt tired and depressed, and had no sex drive at all. I was convinced that it was the beginning of the end for me. Many of my friends with HIV began looking like skeletons due to wasting syndrome, a severe unintentional loss of body weight. And then many died. I was starting to buy into the myth that feeling tired and ending up in bones were normal if one is HIV+.

Luckily in Los Angeles I met HIV+ guys in support groups who were already using testosterone in an underground manner. They boasted about how great they felt and looked. At the time I was terrified to consider the hormone since I had heard that it caused liver and prostate cancer, destroyed one's immune system, and that it would supposedly induce horrible "steroid rage." I was finally convinced to take an educated risk when my fear of dying of wasting became stronger than my fears of testosterone.

I was able to get some testosterone cypionate and had a friend help me inject 200 mg of it in my upper buttock. After two injections (a week apart), I started to improve: My mind was less foggy, my sex drive was returning, my depression lessened, and I started to gain weight. I felt like I was alive again and regained my appetite not only for food, but for life itself. What I thought were symptoms of immune dysfunction were symptoms of having low testosterone. I began to feel like a healthy 34-year old should. With the help of exercise and proper nutrition, I was able to gain 35 pounds of lean body mass, even with uncontrolled HIV virus in my blood. I had hope again.

My amazing transformation inspired me to read all I could about testosterone and androgens in medical journals. This started a journey that has taken me through 16 years of self-education on the subject. In 1999 I co-wrote a book called "Built to Survive: A Comprehensive Guide to the Medical Use of Anabolic Hormones" with Michael Mooney on the medical uses of androgens, exercise, and nutrition to reverse HIV-related wasting and to improve quality of life. After that book was launched, I received many emails from healthy HIV-negative men with questions about testosterone. I realized that the information we gathered in HIV was invaluable also for men without the virus. So I decided to write this book for *all* men who need help, regardless of their health status.

Since its discovery in the early 20ᵗʰ century, the world has learned a lot about testosterone. Unfortunately testosterone is probably also one of the most misunderstood hormones in medicine. Stigma, denial and misconceptions have been barriers for most men to consider its use—even in the presence of all the debilitating symptoms of testosterone deficiency (hypogonadism). These fears have been fueled by a media that equates testosterone supplementation with aggression and with the athletes who abuse it, as well as by physicians who have a poor understanding of testosterone replacement therapy (TRT).

Results from one of the largest studies ever done on testosterone deficiency, the Hypogonadism in Males (HIM) study published in 2006, estimated the overall prevalence of hypogonadism in the United States at approximately 39 percent in men aged 45 years or older. Recent estimates show that 13 million men in the United States may experience testosterone deficiency, although fewer than 10 percent receive treatment for the condition. So why are so many men not receiving treatment for hypogonadism?

Consider that men are known *not* to proactively visit doctors. And consider that the two main symptoms of testosterone deficiency, depression and sexual dysfunction, are topics that most men feel uncomfortable discussing even with their physicians. So even if he is feeling bad enough to finally make it to the doctor, a man is probably more willing to take a physical gut punch than the metaphorical one by admitting out loud that he has problems with his sexual performance or his mood.

Many men suffer needlessly with these problems that dramatically affect their quality of life and how they relate to others. Depression and sexual dysfunction both have been linked to cardiovascular risks factors that affect not only the length of life but more importantly, its quality. Growing older while remaining healthy and independent is surely everyone's wish. This book will provide one of the pieces of the puzzle on how to attain this goal.

Since my last book, several studies have demonstrated that testosterone is an important and relatively safe hormone for those with testosterone deficiency who are monitored by a trained physician. New products like testosterone gels have entered the market and have helped raise testosterone literacy among physicians. But demonization of this hormone and its cousin molecules, anabolic steroids, has not gone away, mostly due to unfounded fears based on lack of information. Regrettably, the media and the U.S.

Congress have focused on the use of testosterone by athletes who utilize these compounds at high doses *without* consulting trained physicians. This media hysteria may also add to the fears about testosterone's side effects present in the minds of potential patients living with hypogonadism who are suffering needlessly and quietly.

Besides researching data on different options, I have purposely tried most of the products that I discuss in this book to provide practical tips on each. I have also been lucky to learn from experiences of many people using these products via my online listserve and lectures in the past 16 years. It is my hope that this book will save readers time and trouble by preventing costly mistakes, wasted time and needless suffering. I tried to write it in accessible language. My suggestions are not intended to be medical advice and I strongly urge every reader to seek the opinion of a qualified and trained physician before engaging in any of the health solutions reviewed in this book.

I have also included valuable information on patient assistance programs and how to find physicians trained in testosterone replacement therapy to save valuable time and money for men searching for solutions to their hypogonadism.

Even though this book focuses on men, you will notice that I included some information about testosterone in women. As of 2010, there is no Food Drug Administration (FDA) approved testosterone product for women, although many doctors have been prescribing small doses in specially compounded creams for lack of libido in females. There are even some products in studies and close to potential approval for women.

Please do not hesitate to email me via my site TestosteroneWisdom.com created to provide updates on new information as it becomes available. Also, please let me know what you think by posting your review on amazon.com.

Wishing you the best health and prosperity,

Nelson Vergel

-2-
Testosterone 101

History of Testosterone

Since man has been walking upright and letting it all hang out, there has been fascination and misinformation about those things that make him male. There were the early beliefs that the eating of penis or testicles from animals was a way to improve virility (still apparently goes on in some parts of the world, given the market for rhino and seal penis). This awareness of the role of the testicles in sexual functioning laid the groundwork for men of science to get involved, sometimes in unusual ways.

In 1889 Charles Edouard Brown-Sequard created a liquid extract made from dog testicles, reporting that it increased his strength. In 1918 Leo L. Stanley transplanted testicles that had been removed from recently executed San Quentin State prisoners into their still living fellow inmates, some of whom claimed improved sexual potency. In the 1920s the French-Russian surgeon Serge Voronoff, made a fortune grafting testicular monkey tissue onto the testicles of aging men.

It wasn't until 1935 that Karoly G. David and Ernst Laqueur isolated crystalline testosterone from testicles. Shortly afterwards, two different groups led by Adolf Butenandt and Leopold Ruzicka developed synthetic methods of preparing testosterone. Butenandt and Ruzicka shared the 1939 Nobel Prize in chemistry for this achievement.

These early formulations of testosterone were quickly broken down in the body. It wasn't until the development of testosterone esters (i.e., a type of chemical compound designed to slow down the breakdown of testosterone in the body) in the 1950s and 1960s that more scientific studies could eventually be done that showed improved muscle mass and strength, libido, energy, bone density, and overall well-being associated with testosterone replacement therapy.

What Is Testosterone and How Does It Work?

Testosterone is synthesized from cholesterol, which, in spite of its bad reputation, is an essential biochemical building block for many hormones and nervous-system molecules. It is the hormone responsible for normal growth and development and maintenance of male sex characteristics. It also affects lean body mass, mood and sexual function in both males and females. It is the primary androgenic (responsible for masculine characteristics) and anabolic (muscle building) hormone.

Testosterone is produced by the testicles in males and by the ovaries in females, with small amounts also produced by the adrenal glands in both genders. Its production and secretion are regulated by other hormones in a hormonal cascade.

As shown in Figure 1, the hormonal and reproductive function of the testicles (gonads) is regulated through interactions among the hypothalamus, the pituitary gland, and the gonads (commonly known as the hypothalamic-pituitary-gonadal axis [HPGA]). The three glands communicate through a cascade of hormones and a self-regulating feedback loop that controls the generation of each hormone. Release of gonadotropin-releasing hormone (GnRH) from the hypothalamus regulates secretion of other hormones (gonadotropins) that influence the testicles by way of the pituitary. GnRH controls the secretion of two gonadotropin hormones- luteinizing hormone (LH) and follicle-stimulating hormone (FSH)- by the anterior pituitary. Luteinizing hormone regulates the production and secretion of testosterone through the Leydig cells of the testes, while FSH stimulates the production of sperm.

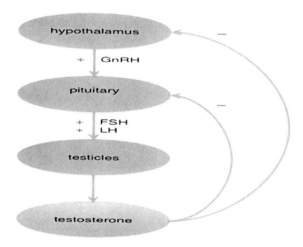

Figure 1. Hormonal cascade that regulates testosterone production in males

When someone is found to have low testosterone blood levels this is
known as "hypogonadism" There are several types of hypogonadism:

- **Primary hypogonadism** is a hypergonadotropic condition (higher
  than normal levels of LH and FSH). This occurs when the testicles
  fail to produce sufficient levels of testosterone to suppress production of LH and FSH. As a result, LH and FSH levels are elevated
  while testosterone levels are decreased. The pituitary gland tries
  to increase testosterone at no avail even after increasing LH and
  FSH.

- **Secondary hypogonadism** results from hypothalamic or pituitary
  dysfunction. It is characterized by disruption of central components
  of the HPGA resulting in decreased levels of GnRH, LH, or FSH.
  In this type of hypogonadism, low levels of LH do not allow for the
  proper stimulation of the production of testosterone by the testes.

- **Mixed hypogonadism** results from a combination of primary and
  secondary causes. The most common cause of mixed hypogonadism
  is late-onset hypogonadism, which occurs with aging. This is
  associated with osteoporosis, decreased lean body mass, reduced
  cognition, fatigue and impairment of libido and erectile function.
  Other causes of mixed hypogonadism include alcoholism, diseases
  (such as uremia, liver failure, AIDS, and sickle cell disease),
  street drugs/alcohol, and medications like corticosteroid steroids
  used for inflammatory conditions. It should be noted that high
  levels of cortisol (hypercortisolism), resulting from either the use
  of anti-inflammatory steroids or physical causes, could lead to
  hypogonadism.

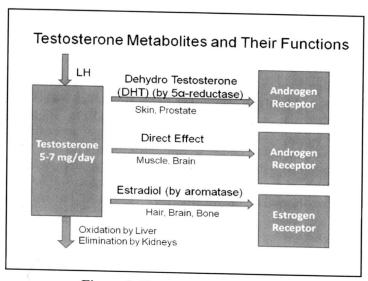

Figure 2. Testosterone Metabolites

As shown in Figure 2, testosterone in the body can convert into other hormones and metabolites. The process in which testosterone is converted into estrogen (a female hormone) by the aromatase enzyme is known as "aromatization". Males with high body fat, aging males, males taking certain medications, males with sex chromosome genetic conditions such as Klinefelters Syndrome or males with a genetic disposition to having higher than normal amounts of aromatase may experience higher conversion of testosterone into estrogen. Estrogen blood levels are usually measured by detecting estradiol, the main estrogen in humans.

Estrogen is a very important hormone for men at the right concentration. It plays an important role in bone, hair, skin, and brain health as well as other functions in men. Large amounts of estrogen can cause mood swings, enlarged breasts (gynecomastia), fat gain, and water retention.

Another metabolite of testosterone is dihydrotestosterone (DHT). DHT has a positive effect on sexual desire but increases the production of excess skin oil, (which can cause acne, hair loss, and prostatic inflammation). So, it is important to monitor and determine the proper dosage of testosterone so that estradiol and DHT are kept within reference ranges needed for healthy body function as well as to prevent unwanted side effects of TRT.

As shown in Figure 3, about 2 percent of the testosterone in the body is active. This "free testosterone" is not attached to binding proteins that would prevent it from interacting with its receptor.

About 40 percent of the body's testosterone is attached to albumin. This is a protein that can release the hormone as the need for it arises in the body. Free testosterone and testosterone attached to albumin are referred to as "bioavailable testosterone".

In a healthy young male, about 60 percent of his testosterone is attached to sex hormone binding globulin (SHBG). Hormones bound to SHBG can't be used by the body and lose their anabolic effect. As males grow older or if illness is present, SHBG sweeps up more and more testosterone, lowering free testosterone and its benefits.

Total testosterone is the sum of bioavailable testosterone and testosterone bound to SHBG. Measuring just the total testosterone in the blood may not provide the whole picture and let you know how much "active" or usable testosterone you have.

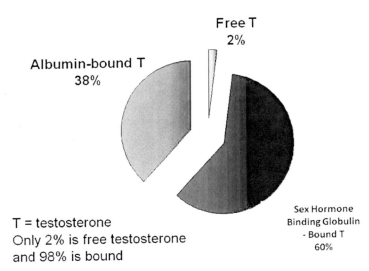

Figure 3. Testosterone fractions in the blood

The normal levels of combined bound and free testosterones in male bodies can range anywhere from 300 to 1,100 ng/dL (nanograms per deciliter). Levels will vary with age and individual factors. It is useful to also measure the level of free testosterone as this may be more indicative of how hormone therapy is progressing. Levels of free testosterone can range between 0.3 and 5 percent of the total testosterone count, with about

2 percent considered an optimal level.

Higher than normal testosterone (i.e., above 1,100 ng/dL of total testosterone) can cause hair loss, acne, mood swings, mania in those with bipolar disorder, water retention, breast enlargement in men, increased aggression and hypersexual behavior, potential prostatic inflammation in older men, increases in the bad cholesterol (low density lipoprotein [LDL]), and decreases in the good cholesterol (high density lipoprotein [HDL]). Like everything in life, balance is key. Too much of a good thing can be detrimental.

Proper monitoring by an experienced physician is extremely important to ensure optimal levels of testosterone, to maximize benefits and to minimize side effects.

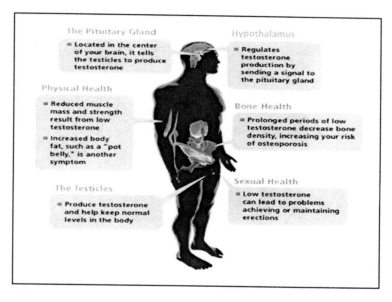

Figure 4. Target organs - beneficial and negative effects of testosterone

What Are the Symptoms of Low Testosterone (Deficiency)?

As mentioned previously, hypogonadism is the medical term for the condition in males that is caused when the body is not producing sufficient amounts of testosterone. What most people don't realize is that in addition to sexual desire, testosterone also affects lean body mass, strength, bone density, mental focus, mood, fat loss, and other important factors in both males and females (Figure 4 shows a male body).

Common complaints for men with hypogonadism include: lower sexual desire (libido), erectile dysfunction (softer erections or lack of erections), depression, low energy and appetite, changes in body composition (lower lean body mass and higher abdominal fat), lower strength, reductions in body and facial hair, less mental focus and decreased height and osteoporosis (decrease in bone density).

As Table 1 shows, normalizing testosterone in people who have lower than normal levels has dramatic benefits, among which are increased sexual desire, lean body mass, bone density, strength, mood, motivation, mental focus, and stamina. However, these benefits can be erased if proper monitoring, dose adjustment, and appropriate choice of testosterone replacement option are not accomplished.

Table 1. Benefits of Normalizing Testosterone

• **Restored sexual desire**
• **Improved erectile function**
• **Improved mood/ sense of wellbeing**
• **Increased lean body mass, strength and stamina**
• **Improved bone density**
• **Decreased fat mass**

Determining If You Have Testosterone Deficiency

In addition to blood tests and physical examination, a brief screening instrument has also been developed by researchers at St. Louis University to aid in the diagnosis of hypogonadism. Known as the Androgen Deficiency in the Aging Male (ADAM) questionnaire:

1. Do you have a decrease in sex drive?
2. Do you lack energy?
3. Have you experienced a decrease in strength and/or endurance?
4. Do you feel shorter? Have you lost height? (Lower bone density can decrease height.)
5. Have you noticed a decreased enjoyment of life?

6. Are you sad and/or grumpy?

7. Are your erections less strong or gone?

8. Has it been more difficult to maintain your erection throughout sexual intercourse?

9. Are you falling asleep after dinner?

10. Has your work performance deteriorated recently?

Other questions that are usually not asked by doctors, but which I've found to be important are the following:

- Are you relating well with people around you?
- Are you being loving to your lover or life partner?
- Are you able to pay attention when someone talks to you?

In my life low testosterone caused problems that went far beyond sex and my body. It affected the way that I related to people and my ability to handle stress at work and in life.

Note that several of the above-mentioned problems can be caused by many other issues unrelated to low testosterone. Depression, anxiety, stress, medications and/or sleep disorders can cause nine of those 10 symptoms (decrease in height would be the only item unrelated to anything but bone loss or back surgery). This questionnaire is not a perfect predictor of low testosterone and should not replace tests for testosterone blood levels.

The benefit of this questionnaire is that it may encourage some men to seek medical advice. Then they can get their testosterone checked and have a physical examination to help determine whether they are indeed hypogonadal.

Causes of Testosterone Deficiency

As discussed before, hypogonadism is caused when the testicles fail to produce normal levels of testosterone. In one type of hypogonadism, testosterone levels are low, while LH and FSH are elevated. In another, there is not enough secretion of LH and FSH needed to tell the testicles to produce needed testosterone.

Some commonly used medications such as Megace (an appetite stimulant), Nizoral (an anti-fungal agent), Prednisone (an anti-inflammatory corticosteroid) and Tagamet (an antacid) can also lower testosterone production. Illness and aging can cause a decrease in testosterone and/or an increase in sex hormone biding globulin (SHBG). Furthermore, high prolactin hormone levels may suggest a pituitary tumor that may be causing a decrease in testosterone production.

It is important that your doctor measure hormones in the HPGA cascade to diagnose what kind of hypogonadism you have. The most common kind of hypogonadism presents low testosterone with normal or elevated FSH and LH levels, which indicates that your testicles are not responding to the signals of both LH and FSH. This is what is called primary hypogonadism.

There are several reasons that testosterone levels may be low:

- Too much testosterone is being converted into estrogen through the activity of the aromatase enzyme, and/or the liver is failing to remove excess estrogen. This could be caused by heavy alcohol intake or the effect of some medications on estrogen clearance in the liver.

- Too much free testosterone is being bound by SHBG. This would be especially apparent if a male's total testosterone level is in the high reference range but his free testosterone (unbound) level is low. As previously mentioned, aging and illness increase SHBG.

- The pituitary gland, which controls testosterone production through the production of LH, is not secreting enough LH to stimulate production of testosterone by the testicles. In this case, total testosterone would be low.

- The hypothalamus is not functioning properly. LH levels of less than 2 ng/mL suggest a lesion in this part of the HPGA.

- The testicles have lost their ability to produce testosterone, despite adequate amounts of LH. In this case, the level of LH would be high (greater than 10 ng/mL) despite a low testosterone level.

- Dehydroepiandrosterone (DHEA) level is abnormally low. DHEA is a hormone produced by the adrenal glands that has a lot of the same benefits as testosterone. It also is a precursor to testosterone in women.

- Disease or infections.

- Street drugs, prescription or over-the-counter medications (more on this later).

- Foods (more on this later).

- Lab error.

- High prolactin levels, which may indicate the presence of a pituitary tumor that impairs production of hormones that tell your testicles to produce testosterone (rare condition but worth mentioning!)

- Defects in genes that affect LH and FSH production.

Diagnosis of Testosterone Deficiency

Lab work will play an important role in diagnosing hypogonadism. Your doctor will likely check your total testosterone and your free testosterone levels. There are some things you should know about these tests, including what they represent and when they should be done.

A "normal" total testosterone scale from most laboratories is generally between 300 and 1,000 ng/dL for men and between 25 and 90 ng/dL for women. The normal range from most laboratories for free testosterone usually is between 3.06 and 24 ng/dL for men and between 0.09 and 1.28 ng/dL for women. Table 2 shows the reference ranges for free testosterone according to age in men.

As mentioned earlier, free testosterone is not bound to blood carrier proteins, so it is "free" to diffuse readily into cells where it signals them to adjust their activity. Some studies report that free testosterone may be a better indicator for quality of life and lean body mass, but there are some conflicting studies on this issue.

Since aging and illness can increase SHBG, which can attach to testosterone to impair its effectiveness, it becomes more important to test for free testosterone if you are older or being challenged by illness.

Measures of free testosterone are controversial. The only standardized and validated method is equilibrium dialysis or by calculating free testosterone levels based on separate measurements of testosterone and SHBG. Other measures of free testosterone are less accurate. So, make sure your doctor is using either one of these methods.

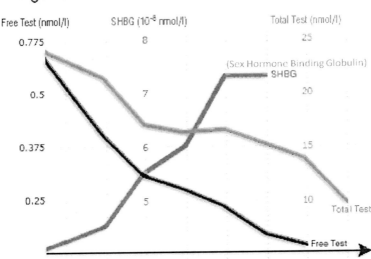

Figure 5. Testosterone decreases as we age as SHBG increases

As you can see in Figure 5, testosterone decreases as we age. This decline is due to many factors that get in the way of retaining a healthy testosterone blood level. Among them are inflammatory states caused by being overweight, diet, medications, alcohol and street drug abuse, stress, lack of adequate sleep, and problems with how the body uses carbohydrates for energy (due to impaired function of the blood sugar controlling hormone insulin). Some experts also think that our own bodies are slowly turning down their engines to get ready for a slower pace and eventual death. However, many physicians in the aging field have now begun to believe that we can grow older while keeping our strength, sexual function, lean tissue, and cognitive function so that we have more "disability-free" years.

Testosterone levels can vary throughout the day. Young and adult men tend to have higher testosterone levels in the morning than in the evening (see Figure 6). This variation is less evident as men age, however. This fact may explain why it's not uncommon for men to have morning erections.

Some physicians recommend doing hormone testing in the morning on an empty stomach, as many things can affect free testosterone measurements, including diet. Elevated insulin caused by eating carbohydrates, for instance, can increase free testosterone levels by reducing plasma levels of SHBG.

Some doctors tend to test this hormone in the late afternoon since the levels may be lower then. In my opinion, it is not practical to restrict testing of this hormone to early morning times and in a fasting state since intraday fluctuations are not that great in men over 30 and it may be equal to laboratory variability.

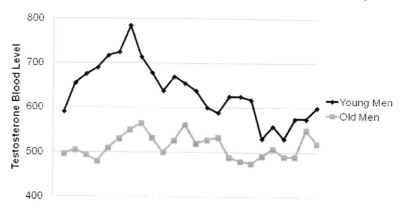

Hourly Testosterone Blood Levels in Healthy Young and Older Men in a Day

Source: Bremner WJ, Vitiello MV, Prinz PN., *J Clin Endocrinol Metab* 1983;56:1278-1281

Figure 6. Variations in testosterone blood levels during the day for young and older men.

Normal values may vary from lab to lab depending on what reference range they use. Your doctor will have your test results in one to two days. Depending on the country, ranges are in nanograms per deciliter (usually in the United States) or nanomoles per liter (Europe and other countries). The conversion factor is:

Testosterone in ng/dL × 0.035 = Testosterone in nanomoles per liter

Table 2. Laboratory Ranges and Codes (courtesy of LabCorp)

Total Testosterone for Males

Age

7 months to 9 years	Less than 30 ng/dL (< 1.04 nmol/L)
10–13 years	1–619 ng/dL (0.04–21.48 nmol/L)
14–15 years	100–540 ng/dL (3.47–18.74 nmol/L)
16–19 years	200–970 ng/dL (6.94–33.66 nmol/L)
20–39 years	270–1,080 ng/dL (9.00–37.48 nmol/L)
40–59 years	350–890 ng/dL (12.15–30.88 nmol/ L)
60 years and older	350–720 ng/dL (12.15–24.98 nmol/L)

Reference Intervals for Free Testosterone

Age

20–29 years old	9.3–26.5 picograms/mililiter (pg/mL)
30–39 years old	8.7–25.1 pg/mL
40–49 years old	6.8–21.5 pg/mL
50–59 years old	7.2–24.0 pg/mL

A Note about Saliva Testing (from Aetna Insurance Company)

Salivary tests of estrogen, progesterone, testosterone, melatonin, cortisol and DHEA have become available to consumers over the Internet. Some of these websites include a questionnaire to allow consumers to determine whether they need saliva testing, and a form that allows consumers to order these tests online. The results of these tests are purportedly used to determine the need prescriptions of DHEA, vitamins, herbs, phytoestrogens, and other anti-aging regimens.

The medical literature on salivary testing correlates salivary levels with serum levels, the gold standard measurement. However, the medical literature fails to demonstrate that salivary tests are appropriate for screening, diagnosing, or monitoring patients with menopause, osteoporosis, or other consequences of aging.

According to a committee opinion by the American College of

Obstetricians and Gynecologists (ACOG, 2005), salivary hormone level testing used by proponents to 'tailor' hormone therapy isn't meaningful because salivary hormone levels vary within each woman depending on her diet, the time of day, the specific hormone being tested, and other variables.

An assessment by the Institute for Clinical Systems Improvement (2006) concluded: "Currently, there is insufficient evidence in the published scientific literature to permit conclusions concerning the use of salivary hormone testing for the diagnosis, treatment or monitoring of menopause and aging."

The North American Menopause Society (2005) has concluded: "Salivary testing is not considered to be a reliable measure of testosterone levels."

Flyckt and colleagues (2009) compared salivary versus serum measurements of total testosterone (TT), bioavailable testosterone (BT; consisting of free testosterone [FT] and albumin-bound testosterone), and FT from samples collected simultaneously in women who were either receiving transdermal testosterone patch supplementation (300 micrograms/d) or a placebo patch. Naturally and surgically post-menopausal women receiving concomitant hormone therapy were recruited to participate in a 24- to 52-week phase III trial of a 300 micrograms/day transdermal testosterone patch for the treatment of hypoactive sexual desire disorder. Initial analysis demonstrated high correlations between TT, BT, and FT levels ($r = 0.776$ to 0.855). However, there was no correlation with salivary testosterone levels for any of the serum testosterone subtypes ($r = 0.170$ to 0.261). After log transformation, salivary testosterone correlated modestly with BT ($r = 0.436$, $p < 0.001$), FT ($r = 0.452$, $p < 0.001$), and TT ($r = 0.438$, $p < 0.001$). The authors concluded that although salivary testing of testosterone concentrations is an appealing alternative because it is inexpensive and non-invasive, these findings do not support the routine use of salivary testosterone levels in post-menopausal women.

Gröschl (2008) provided an overview of the current applications of salivary hormone analysis. The author noted that although saliva has not yet become a mainstream sample source for hormone analysis, it has proven to be reliable and, in some cases, even superior to other body fluids. Nevertheless, much effort will be needed for this approach to receive acceptance over the long-term, especially by clinicians. Such effort entails the development of specific and standardized analytical tools, the establishment of defined reference intervals, and implementation of round-robin trials. One major obstacle is the lack of compliance sometimes observed in outpatient saliva donors. Moreover, the author stated that there is a need for standardization of both collection and analysis methods in order to attain better comparability and evaluation of published salivary hormone data.

Testosterone Replacement Options

Top Mistakes People Make When Taking Testosterone Replacement Therapy

I have heard of so many mistakes being made by people taking testosterone replacement therapy. Some mistakes seriously impacted their quality of life, or resulted in men stopping testosterone prematurely. Here are a few of the biggest errors that I've witnessed:

1. **Using "street sources" of testosterone:** I have met many men whose doctors do not support their use of testosterone, so they buy it on the black market or from some guy at their gyms. This is illegal. Testosterone is classified as a controlled substance under the Anabolic Steroids Control Act of 1990 and has been assigned to Schedule III. It is regulated by the Drug Enforcement Agency (DEA). A doctor can legally prescribe it but it is illegal to use without a prescription. Be aware that the buying or the using of testosterone without a proper prescription may have legal consequences. The use of testosterone and its cousin molecules (anabolic steroids) is illegal in the United States for those without a medical diagnosis that justifies their use (e.g. anemia, wasting, and hypogonadism). If after reading this book you still decide to get testosterone in the black market, be beware that you could be set up by informants who may alert the DEA of your purchase. Also, importing testosterone even if you have a prescription is not legal. In a nut shell: only use testosterone after a physician gives you a prescription and do not import it from other countries.

   The use of "street" testosterone is also dangerous. No one knows what those products may contain. Some so-called testosterone products may simply contain peanut, sesame or grape-seed oil. You also run the risk of exposure to contaminants that could cause infection.

Not having a doctor follow-up your blood work is a sure way to get in trouble! If you have low testosterone, there are hundreds of doctors who will prescribe testosterone replacement therapy (refer to the Appendix section for directories). If you are using testosterone to increase muscle mass or to improve athletic performance even though you have normal testosterone levels, be smart and research all you can. And please, read the information in this book about how stopping testosterone can cause health problems (if you are using black market testosterone, chances are that your source will eventually run out).

2. **Not exploring what testosterone option is best for you**: Since there is an assortment of options for testosterone replacement, it's important that you take the time to really find out what's best for you. Several factors are involved in deciding what would be the best testosterone replacement option for you. Among them are cost, insurance coverage, convenience, preference for daily versus weekly use, lack of time to stick to a strict daily schedule, fears of needles, and physician familiarity of the different products. For instance, some health management organizations (HMOs) programs only pay for testosterone injections since they are the cheapest option. However some men have needle-phobia and dislike weekly or bi-weekly injections that may require them to go see their doctors that frequently (some doctors do not teach their patients to self inject at home). Other men are prescribed daily gels even if their busy lives make it difficult to be perfectly compliant to the daily therapy. Some men without insurance or financial means decide not to seek help since they do not know that there are patient assistance programs set up by manufacturers, or the fact that compounding pharmacies can make cheap gels and creams with a doctor prescription (details on this information is available in the Appendix section). Every testosterone option has advantages and disadvantages that may be more suitable for one person over another, so read the following section on treatment options.

3. **Not using the right dose:** Men who start testosterone need to have their testosterone blood levels rechecked two weeks or one month after they start therapy (depending on the testosterone formulation), right before they administer the corresponding dose for that day or week. This is critical since these results are essential

to deciding if the dose is right for you. Total testosterone blood levels less than 500 ng/dL that are not improving your sexual desire and energy should be increased to 500 to 1,000 ng/dL by increasing the frequency of injection or the dose. Some doctors fail to retest after they get a patient started on testosterone since they assume most men respond to 200 mg bi-weekly injections or 5 grams per day of gels. The reality is that many men require higher doses to reach total testosterone levels above mid range of normal. Those men tend to stop testosterone early because they perceive no benefits at "average" doses. Incorrect frequency of injections is a common mistake and is actually worse than not getting treatment at all. See the next sections for more details on this.

4.   **Cycling on and off testosterone:** Testosterone replacement is a life-long commitment in most cases. Once you start you should assume that you will stay on it unless you have an unmanageable side effect. Some patients think that "giving the body a break" once every few weeks is a good thing. What they do not know is that during the time that you are taking testosterone, your testicles stop producing it. When you stop replacement therapy you are left with *no* testosterone in your system for weeks while your HPG hormonal axis normalizes. Depression, weight loss, lack of motivation, and loss of sex drive can appear rapidly and with a vengeance. A few men never have their hormonal axis return to normal after stopping testosterone (especially if they were hypogonadal at baseline). Read more details on this in the section entitled "HPGA dysfunction."

5.   **Stopping testosterone abruptly due to an unrelated problem:** Some of us may be taking medications for other conditions along with testosterone. Sometimes new medications can increase cholesterol and triglycerides and/or liver enzymes. Some doctors prematurely blame testosterone instead of the new medications that someone might have started. I have seen people suffer because of this poor judgment of their doctors. Weeks later, they learn that stopping testosterone did not improve any of these problems but by then they feel tired, depressed, and asexual.

6.   **Not knowing how to manage potential side effects:** Luckily, this will not happen to you after you finish reading this book. I know men who stopped testosterone due to swelling in their nipple area.

acne, moodiness, perceived lack of benefit, hair loss, or a prostatic specific antigen (PSA) increase that was due to a prostatic infection. Knowing how to manage these side effects is essential to long-term success. If you know what side effects may occur and how to deal with them, you are less likely to prematurely stop therapy. You may just need to readjust the dose, change the delivery method, or take a medication to counteract the potential problem. Only the best physicians, who do not overreact to a side effect, know how to do this.

7. **Having a life style that is not "testosterone friendly":** If you smoke, drink more than two drinks a day, smoke too much pot, are overweight, do not exercise, do not keep your blood sugar or lipids in control, and do not show up to doctor's appointments, you do not have a testosterone-friendly lifestyle. Studies have shown that these factors may influence your sexual function and long-term health. Excessive alcohol can decrease testosterone. Exercise can increase it if done properly or decrease it if overdone. You can read more about this later in this book.

8. **Not reading or staying "networked" with other patients:** Being in isolation about information makes you a less effective patient. There are online groups of men who discuss testosterone and other issues (see the Resource section). Sharing your experiences and learning from others are keys to being an empowered and proactive patient. It's the only way to maximize the benefits of any therapy you are using. Many of the practical "tricks" that I have learned have been obtained via this method. The collective wisdom of other people with similar issues is more powerful than just relying on everything your doctor tells, or does not tell you. Besides, most doctors treat educated patients a lot better than those who are timid about sharing and asking questions.

9. **Not switching doctors when you have to:** Changing doctors can be difficult, especially if you are not a networked patient who reads a lot about your condition. Many people do not have options and have to see a certain doctor in a health management organization (HMO) setting. But most of us have the option of searching for educated doctors who are not condescending and who treat you as an equal. Your doctor should be your partner in your health and not just an unquestioned authority. Although they are saving lives and

have spent hundreds of hours in school and practice to do so, they are human beings who are exposed to myths and misconceptions similar to ours. I have heard the most irrational things from doctors about testosterone replacement that make me question how unfortunate their patients may be. Be sure to do your homework and find a doctor who supports *you* in your search for optimum health. See the Resource section for directories of physicians who are trained in testosterone replacement management.

10. **Poor compliance:** Forgetting when to inject or apply gels is a common complaint. Good time management and reminders are extremely important. Find reminders that work for you. I use Google calendar which can be set up to send me text messages to my phone as reminders. Avoid the yo-yo effect that poor compliance causes! Testosterone replacement is a lifetime and life style commitment that should be explored with care.

Testosterone Formulations

In theory testosterone replacement should approximate the body's own natural production of the hormone. The average male produces 4 to 7 mg of testosterone a day with plasma levels in early morning and lower levels in the evening. Women produce around a 12th of those rates.

Testosterone replacement is usually a life-long commitment. It is a decision that should not be made without a discussion with your health care provider. Starting and stopping testosterone can have negative effects on someone's quality of life (more on this topic later).

There are testosterone replacement products that require daily dosing (orals, buccal, and gels), once a week or two weeks dosing (injections), and once every three- to four-month dosing (long-acting testosterone undecanoate injections not yet approved in the United States as of 2011) or testosterone pellets).

Males who are hypogonadal can be given continuous testosterone replacement therapy in a wide assortment of ways. These include:

1. Oral capsules

2. Testosterone injections

3. Transdermal (absorbed through the skin) testosterone cream or gel

4. Transdermal testosterone patch

5. Buccal (sublingual and gum adherent)

6. Pellets (that are implanted subcutaneously)

Oral Agents

Oral testosterone formulations are quickly absorbed by the liver and therefore require relatively large doses. Because of the risk of liver toxicity they are rarely prescribed. Do not waste your money or time using oral testosterone. Also, avoid over-the-counter supplements that claim to increase testosterone. Most do *not* increase testosterone for more than a few minutes and can also affect your liver and blood pressure. Oral testosterone also seems to cause larger decreases of the good cholesterol (HDL) than other forms of testosterone therapies.

Chemically unbound testosterone, if taken orally, is immediately deactivated by the liver. Two chemically modified forms of testosterone are available that require several doses a day: methyl testosterone and testosterone undecanoate (not approved in the United States but popular in Canada).

Methyl testosterone

Methyl testosterone is one of the earliest available oral testosterones. Its chemical structure is the hormone testosterone with an added methyl group at the c-17 alpha position of the molecule to slow down its clearance by the liver. The use of oral c-17 alpha methylated testosterone causes toxicity to the liver and is not recommended for testosterone hormone therapy. Brand names around the world include "Metesto," "Methitest," "Testred," "Oreton Methyl," and "Android." These products are responsible for many of the misconceptions that still exist about testosterone replacement due to their liver and lipid problems. The same information is applicable to fluroxymesterone, another oral formulation no longer used in the United States.

Testosterone undecanoate

Testosterone undecanoate is not a c-17 alpha alkylated hormone. Therefore it is considered a safer oral form of testosterone. It is designed to be absorbed through the small intestine into the lymphatic system, and has fewer negative effects on the liver. Brand names around the world for oral testosterone undecanoate include "Andriol," "Androxon," "Understor," "Restandol," and "Restinsol." It is not available in the United States but widely used in Canada and some European countries.

One disadvantage of orally administered undecanoate is that it is eliminated from the body very quickly, usually within three to four hours. Frequent administration is necessary—usually from three to six capsules a day, which makes it impractical for most men with busy lives.

PERSONAL COMMENT: I've never used oral testosterones and I never will. Other formulations are so much more user-friendly.

Intramuscular Injections

The most common testosterone replacement used by men worldwide is intramuscular testosterone injection. It's also the oldest and most economical way to increase blood levels of testosterone. This most cost effective option is usually covered by insurance programs and community clinics.

The two most common esters, testosterone cypionate and testosterone enanthate, are both generic medications in the United States. They are given at a weekly dose of about 100 to 200 mg a week (or 200 to 300 mg every two weeks).

Currently, a 10 ml bottle of 200 mg/ml (2000 total milligrams per bottle) of testosterone cypionate obtained in U.S. pharmacies cost around $85-$115. The cost of the same strength and amount of testosterone cypionate costs $33- $50 from compounding pharmacies. It is the same product, so if your insurance company does not pay for testosterone, make sure that you use compounding pharmacies. More information on compounding will be provided later.

Some physicians have patients come to their office for injections and others empower their patients to do so at home. A minority of physicians charges a fee for the office visit when you come for an injection, which can increase your costs.

When you get a prescription for any testosterone ester, make sure that it is for a 10-ml vial, not 1-ml vial. In the U.S., 1-ml vials are available but they are usually more expensive and not very practical. Many physicians will write an open-ended prescription that will look like this:

1. *Testosterone Cypionate (or Depo Testosterone), 10 ml, 200mg/ml, #1, as directed, 1 refill*

Others will write:

2. *Testosterone Cypionate, 10 ml, 200 mg/ml, #1, 200 mg q 2 weeks, 1 refill*

Or
3. Testosterone Cypionate , 10 ml, 200 mg/ml #1, 100 mg q 1 week, 1 refill

Be sure your physician gives you a more flexible prescription that reads like my first example. This type of prescription will provide room for you to adjust the dosage during the first two months as well as get a refill whenever you need it.

Optimum testosterone doses can range from 100 mg to 300 mg a week but it is practically impossible to predict an individual's response. Giving yourself a little room for adjustment keeps you from running out of testosterone if your insurance company denies your next refill because they think it's too early. Of course, your physician has to ensure that your dose is adjusted based on your total or free testosterone blood levels.

When using injectable testosterone, your doctor will want to measure your total blood testosterone levels right before your next injection after the first month (it takes a while for the blood levels to stabilize). If testosterone is >900 ng/dl (24.5 nmol/liter) or < 500 ng/dl, adjust dose or frequency. Anecdotally, most men seem to need to have total testosterone levels above 500 ng/dl (mid point of normal range) to experience any of the expected sexual function benefits.

A dose for women is anywhere from 2.4 to 20 mg/week but because it is difficult to inject such low doses and because of the risk of masculinization (growth or facial hair, deepening of the voice, and growth of clitoris), many doctors prefer low dose creams to treat women. Compounding pharmacies like Women's International Pharmacy can guide doctors on how to test and prescribe testosterone gels to women. Their website is womensinternational.com. They have an excellent information packet that they send to people for free that contains several research papers and protocols for women.

There is no commercially available FDA-approved testosterone therapy for women in the United States as of 2011, but one option may be approved in 2012 (Libigel, mentioned later). However, many doctors can legally prescribe testosterone to women in an off-label manner using compounded gels and creams. However, some doctors are reluctant to prescribe any hormones to women since the discouraging results from female hormone replacement in women showed increased cardiovascular risk in women. For a great articles and books on women and hormones, I highly recommend Dr. Susan Rako's page: www.susanrako.com/workshop.htm

Injections have the advantage of once-per-week (or every two weeks) administration, so it may be a more acceptable option for men who do not want to deal with the daily administration typically needed with gels. However there are concerns about their "peak-and-valleys" testosterone blood level patterns.

As you can see in Figures 7 and 8, 200 mg testosterone injections currently used in the United States produce an unnaturally high blood testosterone level during the initial few days after an injection. Then the blood level drops off each day and falls to baseline in about 10 days. This method does not effectively deliver sustained normal blood levels of testosterone or mimic the natural daily pattern of testosterone release as well as other treatment options. There is a concern that some men using 200 mg of testosterone cypionate every two weeks may have low levels of testosterone by day 10, so they spend four days with low testosterone before their next injection. For this reason, I have seen that a dose of 100 mg of testosterone cypionate or enanthate weekly is becoming more and more commonly prescribed by doctors who treat a lot of hypogonadal men.

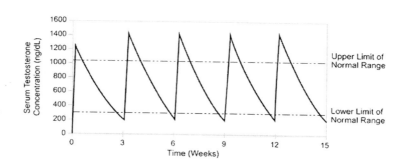

Behre HM et al. In: *Testosterone: Action. Deficiency. Substitution.* Berlin, Germany: Springer-Verlag; 1998:329-348

Figure 7.

**200 mg of Testosterone Enanthate Injections Every Two Weeks in 33 men age 22-65
Effect on Total and Bioavailable Testosterone, Estradiol, and DHT**

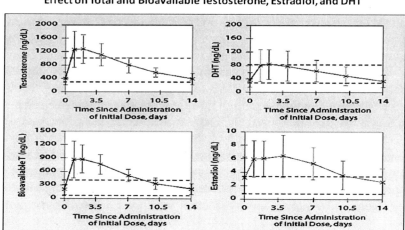

Adapted from Dobs AS, et al.. *J Clin Endocrinol Metab.* 1999;84:3469–3478.

Figure 8. Blood testosterone, estradiol and DHT concentration curves
after a 200 mg injection of testosterone enanthate every two weeks

Your doctor should re-check your testosterone level after one month
(after steady state occurs) right before the next injection. This testing
schedule allows him to see whether normal levels are still present when
you reach your lowest testosterone blood level. If serum total testosterone
level is more than 900 ng/dL or less than 500 ng/dL right before the next dose,
he /she can adjust the dose or the frequency accordingly.

Due to testosterone's effect as a stimulant of red blood cell production, injections produce unusually strong stimulation during the first peak
days. This appears to increase the potential for elevated hemoglobin and
hematocrit indicating that you have too many red blood cells. These can
increase your cardiovascular risks. Creams, gels, and patches appear to be
less likely to produce this side effect, though study results are conflicting.

Anecdotally I hear that injections promote elevations in blood pressure
more than creams, gel, and patches. It also appears that the effect on
brain chemistry and the nervous system that might promote increased
assertiveness can be stronger with injections. There will be more discussion
on this subject later. But I would love to see head-to-head comparison
studies between testosterone injections and gels, since none have been
performed to date. Hopefully, with the potential approval of Aveed (a

longer acting testosterone ester) in the future, its manufacturer would be compelled to do such a study to convince insurance companies that their product may be more cost effective and less problematic than the daily gels currently approved in the United States (Androgel and Testim) or the weekly or bi-weekly injections that many men are currently using.

I have met some men that have switched from injections to gels and then eventually switch back to injections. It seems that they need the higher level of overall metabolic stimulation that injectable testosterone provides. Usually, those men also say they feel very little improvement with the use of gels or creams. They also usually prefer the convenience of an injection every one or two weeks to the daily administration of a gel. And, unlike gels, injections have no potential risk of transferring testosterone through skin contact with other people.

Injectable testosterone has also shown to increase blood levels of testosterone and DHT in proportion with the dose. But gels seem to increase DHT a lot more than the expected increase due to higher testosterone, so some men with benign prostatic inflammation may prefer injections than gels. The mechanism for this observation may be based on the fact that they may be more DHT receptors in the skin layers, but no one has really proven this fact.

As you can see, there is no one-size-fits-all approach that works for everyone. Blank statements about one option being better than other have to be done in the context of other factors that go beyond the obvious. Convenience, doctor's prescription habits, personal life style, cost, and what your insurance company pays are factors that determine what you use.

It is important to follow a strict injection procedure (for helpful tips, see the section on How to Inject Testosterone Safely). Some men report soreness in the injection area and experience coughing spells after injecting. In rare cases, some men have had infections in the injection site due to unsanitary techniques!

Commonly Used Injectable Esters for Testosterone Replacement Therapy

Testosterone esters are modifications made to the testosterone molecule to increase the time the liver breaks it down, so that you do not have to inject every day. Esters consist of the actual testosterone molecule, with a carbon chain attached to it. This carbon chain controls something called the partition co-efficient, which translates into how soluble the drug will be once in the bloodstream. Also, the larger the carbon chain, the longer the ester, the less soluble the drug is in water, and the longer it stays in your body. Also, additions to the basic testosterone molecule make it harder for the liver to break it down, which also increases the time testosterone stays in your system (a good thing since we do not want to deal with injections too frequently).

There are several types of testosterone esters: testosterone cypionate, enanthate, propionate, or undecanoate. Outside the United States, there is a product with a combination of the first three esters that is called Sustanon 250 (250 mg of a mixture of cypionate, enanthate, and propionate). Since every ester may have slightly different blood level decay after administration, it is speculated that this combination may allow better distribution of testosterone blood levels in 14 days. Sustanon is not available in the United States but compounding pharmacies may customize similar formulations.

Testosterone cypionate, enanthate, or other ester is injected slowly into the muscle of the buttock where it forms a reservoir of the hormone. Then testosterone is gradually released from the reservoir into the blood stream. There is usually a peak concentration in the blood within the first two days and then a gradual decrease to baseline. Everyone is different and the rate of decrease of blood levels tends to change depending on body weight, fat content, activity level, medications, illness, and liver metabolism.

Testosterone Enanthate

Testosterone enanthate is one of the main forms of testosterone prescribed to men in the United States. It is a slow-acting ester, with a release time between 8 and 10 days. The name brand of testosterone enanthate available in the United States is called "Delatestryl," which is suspended in sesame oil. Testosterone enanthate is typically injected once every week to once every two weeks. Generic testosterone enanthate can also be obtained through a compounding pharmacy; such pharmacies can mix the enanthate in either sesame, grape seed or cottonseed oil. Some mix different esters for patients since this may give better blood level distribution, although no studies have been done in the United States using ester blends.

For more details about this product, refer to the Appendix section for the package insert. Package inserts are required by the FDA to be provided with every product when you pick it up at the pharmacy. They are also required when magazine ads or promotional materials are provided on products. That is why I thought it would be a good idea to include a package insert on an injectable and a gel at the end of this book. Every patient should read package inserts of every medication they take, but keeping in mind that a lot of the side effects listed are not common and only happen in special circumstances. But it does not hurt to know them just in case!

Testosterone cypionate

Testosterone cypionate is the other main injectable form of testosterone prescribed to men in the United States. It is a slow-acting ester with a release time of 8 to 10 days, similar to that of enanthate. The name brand available in the United States is called "Depo-Testosterone," which is suspended in cottonseed oil. Testosterone cypionate is typically injected anywhere from once every week to once every two weeks. Some doctors like to prescribe 300 mg every three weeks, but I believe that really accentuates the peaks and valleys of testosterone blood levels a lot more than the most commonly used dose of 100 or 200 mg every two weeks. Cheaper generic testosterone cypionate can also be obtained through a compounding pharmacy which can mix it in either sesame, grape seed or cotton seed oil.

Sustanon 100 or 250

"Sustanon" is the brand name for two formulas of injectable testosterone that contain a blend of esters. "Sustanon 100" contains 100 mg of three testosterone esters: testosterone propionate, testosterone phenyl propionate, and testosterone isocaproate. "Sustanon 250" contains a total of 250 mg of four testosterone esters: testosterone propionate, testosterone phenyl propionate, testosterone isocaproate, and testosterone decanoate. Both formulas feature fast-acting and slow-acting esters, and can be injected anywhere from once every week to once every four weeks. Sustanon is prescribed outside the United States, but a formulation similar to it can be compounded legally by compounding pharmacies since all of its esters are available in the United States.

Other Injectcable Esters of Testosterone

Testosterone propionate

Testosterone propionate is a fast-acting ester with a release time of three to four days. To keep blood levels from fluctuating greatly, propionate is usually injected from one to three times a week. It is for this reason that it is not usually prescribed that much. Some users also report that propionate is a more painful injection, with swelling and noticeable pain around the injection site.

Testosterone phenyl propionate

Testosterone phenyl propionate is a slow-acting ester, with a release time of one to three weeks. A popular name brand for T-phenyl propionate is "Testolent." Testosterone phenyl propionate is also one of the components of Sustanon.

Testosterone Undecanoate

Testosterone undecanoate injections are known as the brand name Nebido around the world. In the United States it will be called Aveed. Aveed is currently under review for approval by the FDA. This ester may stay longer in your system so that less frequent injections may be needed. The injection is usually given once every 10 to 14 weeks, though the frequency will depend on your individual testosterone levels. After your first injection you may be asked to come back for another injection at week six. For use in the United States, the company claims that only five injections a year are needed (compared to 48 injections per year for a 100 mg per week regimen). In other countries, a large injection dose of 1000 mg are allowed. The FDA did not allow the manufacturer to use this dose in studies done in this country due to fears of side effects.

In an open-label study which enrolled 130 hypogonadal men with blood total testosterone levels below 300 ng/dL at study entry, Aveed was dosed as an intramuscular injection (750 mg) at baseline, at week four, and then every 10 weeks throughout the remainder of the 21-month study. Approximately 70 percent of patients completed all injections and 94 percent of them had total testosterone from 300 to 1,000 nanograms/ml through the entire study.

After Nebido was approved in Europe a small number of European patients experienced respiratory symptoms immediately following an intramuscular injection of 1000 mg in a 4 cc injection volume, (versus the 750 mg, 3 cc injection volume used in the United States). The makers of Nebido believe, and the FDA concurs, that the reaction is likely the result of a small amount of the oily solution immediately entering the vascular system from the injection site. This known yet uncommon complication of oil-based depot injections may be related to inappropriate injection technique or site.

The problem is characterized by short-term reactions involving an urge to cough or a shortness of breath. In some rare cases the reaction had been classified as serious or the patient had experienced other symptoms such as dizziness, flushing or fainting. In U.S. clinical trials of Nebido 750 mg (3 cc injection volume), the proposed dose in the U.S., there was a single, mild, non-serious case of oil-based coughing.

The U.S. manufacturer, Endo Pharmaceuticals, is gathering data to address concerns about the respiratory symptoms. It is not known how much longer it will take the get this product approved in the United States as of June 2010. And even if it gets approved, it may not be widely available for people to buy through private health insurance if the company decides to price it as high as gels.

PERSONAL COMMENT: I have used testosterone enanthate, cypionate, and Sustanon 250. I cannot say I can tell the difference in the way I felt. I also tried one injection of Nebido in Mexico. After a big injection of the recommended dose of 1,000 mg, my testosterone blood levels remained above 450 ng/ml for four and a half months; my mood and stamina remained very good throughout. It was nice not having to worry about remembering to inject every week.

How to Inject Testosterone Safely

Some men prefer testosterone injections because of the convenient dosing and/or they report feeling much better when using injections versus gels. Sometimes their insurance companies only pay for injections. Men without health insurance also tend to use injections since they are a lot cheaper than gels. If your doctor empowers you to self-inject at home, it will be more convenient and possible cheaper (some physicians charge for the office visit). I tell men that they can always switch from gels to injections and vice versa depending on what they learn as they optimize their testosterone replacement.

So you've decided to go with injectable testosterone. Your decision may arise out of your realization that you won't remember to make daily use of the gels. It may have made the choice because your insurance company refuses to pay for anything but the injectable. If your doctor is letting you self-inject there are some things for you to know:

- **Keep it safe.** Sharing used needles with another person is a definite no. And this goes for the syringes too. You can contract all kinds of diseases including hepatitis B and C, and HIV. Doctors give you a prescription for syringes and needles for a reason. There is no need to risk ruining your health. Don't even think about re-using your own syringes and needles. Unclean needles and syringes can cause infections. Buy a "sharps" container and put your used needles and syringes in it. These containers are available at most pharmacies. Those using underground testosterone usually have the most difficult time trying to find syringes since pharmacies won't provide supplies without a prescription. .

- **Keep it moving.** Try not to inject into the exact same area more than twice a month. Vigorously massage the area after you've injected. This helps reduce pain.

- **Keep it clean**. Wash your hands before starting. Clean the area to be injected using an alcohol swab. Clean the top of the testosterone vial with an alcohol swab before you insert the needle to draw the product. The alcohol swabs are available at most pharmacies and do not require a prescription.

- **Keep it sharp**. Use a new needle every time. I personally like using smaller gauge needles (18 gauge, 1 inch) which are bigger in size, to draw the testosterone from the bottle. I then use a new larger gauge needle, which is smaller in size (23 gauge, 1 inch) when injecting. The reason for this is that after a needle is used once, it loses its sharpness. Injections with dull needles hurt a lot more. I ask the pharmacist to sell me several 18 gauge needles without syringes for drawing the testosterone, plus the same number of 23 gauge, 1 inch, 3 ml syringes. Some doctors think that it is difficult to inject through a thin needle of this size, but I have done it for years without any such problems. I would rather take a little longer injecting than having to endure pain caused by using a thicker needle.

- What to look for before injecting.
  - **Expiration dates**
    - Check the expiry dates of every product.
  - **Waste**
    - Make sure that contaminated waste is disposed of safely. Ask your pharmacist to sell you a plastic sharps container.

- **Materials needed**
  Vial with required testosterone, 20-23 gauge syringe with a capacity of 3 ml and a needle length of 1-1.5 inches, an extra 18 gauge needle for drawing testosterone into syringe, two alcohol swabs.

Guide to Injecting Testosterone:
1. Wash your hands (with a disinfectant/anti-bacterial soap).
2. Layout your vial of testosterone, needle and/or syringe, alcohol wipes and tissue on a clean surface (e.g. a clean towel, paper towel, etc).
3. Sit down and get comfy.

4. Change the 23 gauge needle that comes with the syringe for a 18 gauge one for drawing testosterone from the vial. Set aside the 23 gauge needle for injecting later.
5. Unseat/loosen the cap from the needle. Leave the cap on loose until ready to draw the testosterone. Remember not to touch the needle!
6. Wipe off the "nipple" on the top of the vial with an alcohol wipe.
7. Remove the cap of the needle without touching the needle or the needle touching anything. Draw around 1 cc of air into the syringe by pulling back on the plunger.
8. Up-end the testosterone vial.
9. Insert the needle through the center of the neoprene nipple.
10. With the needle tip immersed in the fluid, slowly depress the plunger, pushing all of the air into the oil (you'll see the bubbles).
11. After all the air is out of the syringe, slowly pull back on the plunger until the proper amount of testosterone is drawn into the syringe. (Not everyone's dosage is the same. Check your prescription or consult with your physician or pharmacist for the correct amount. Some will inject more than 1 cc, some less.)
12. You may need to "pump" the plunger to get a complete fill. As long as you don't remove the needle, you can let the fluid go in and out as much as needed.
13. When you have the correct amount in the syringe, gently pull the needle out of the vial.
14. Draw a small amount of air into the syringe—one very small bubble.
15. Slip the needle back into the cap if you want to take a break before injecting. (It's really important not to touch the needle itself at any point.)
16. Change the needle to a 23 gauge one
17. Pick an injection site on your thigh or buttocks (see Figure 9). You'll want to alternate sites, so remember which site you last injected. For your thigh, target the spot by placing one hand just about at your knee and the other at your hip—the area in between is pretty much fair game. The best area is the outer part of the quad, so stay to the outside of the midline of your thigh, but not too far to the outside/underside. The buttocks is slightly more tricky—both to reach and to isolate the exact spot. Talk to your physician or nurse about the exact location.

Nelson Vergel

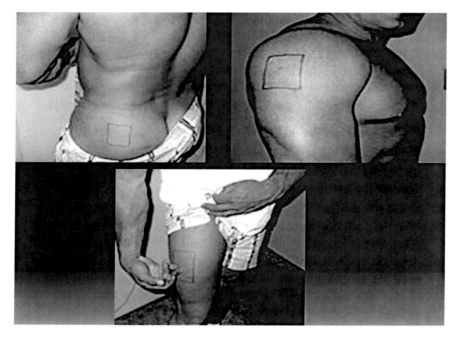

Figure 9. Testosterone injection sites

18. Clean the injection site with an alcohol wipe. Wipe in a circular motion, to a circumference of about two inches surrounding the injection site. Allow the skin to dry to prevent the alcohol from being introduced into the muscle as the needle is inserted, causing pain or burning. Remember not to touch the area just cleansed with the alcohol wipe.

19. Uncap the needle—remember not to touch the needle or the swabbed area on your thigh. The air bubble should be near the plunger end of the syringe.

20. Go to it and stick it in! Fast or slow, either is fine. Pierce the skin at a 90 degree angle. It must go through the subcutaneous tissue/fatty tissue and deep into the muscle.

21. If using a 1" needle, stop about 1/8" from the base; if using a 1.5" needle, stop about 1/4" from the base. (This is true for average-sized bodies. Talk with your physician about the appropriate needle length for your body.)

22. After the needle has been inserted, aspirate by holding the barrel of the syringe steady with your non dominant hand and by pulling back on the plunger with your dominant hand. You'll see some air bubbles in the testosterone. If there's just air/clear fluid—no

blood—then it's ok to proceed. If there is blood, either push the needle in or pull the needle back a little and pull back on the plunger again, or pull the needle out and start over.

23. Holding the syringe steady, inject the testosterone steadily and <u>slowly</u> by depressing the plunger until all of the testosterone is injected. The air bubble in the syringe should follow the testosterone and will "pack" the testosterone down into your muscle. There will be a slight "pop" as the bubble leaves the syringe.

24. Pull the needle out—again, slow or fast depending upon your preference. (I think it's usually best to pull out slow. Sometimes the injection site may bleed a little when you withdraw the needle, just be prepared to apply some gentle pressure with some clean tissue(s).

25. Slide the needle back into the cap. (Remember DO NOT reseat the cap by pressing the tip of the cap towards the needle's point.)

26. Dispose of your needles properly in what is known as a sharps container (i.e., a needle disposal container).

Once you inject a few times, you should lose begin to lose your fear of injecting. You can also have your partner or good friend inject you if you do not feel comfortable doing so. Your doctor's medical staff can help you develop your technique.

PERSONAL COMMENT: I think I have great injection technique using my upper glutes but I have experienced the post-injection cough. It is a strange feeling compared to inhaling very cold air that makes you cough and feel out of breath for a few minutes. This probably has happened to me only five times in 16 years of testosterone use When it has happened I find that breathing quickly into a paper bag helps it go away faster. Honestly, I cannot tell you if I used a different injection site since I always use the upper buttock area close to my hip. By the way, I hate injecting in my legs since I think it hurts a lot more and the potential for problems is greater. But some men do not feel comfortable or capable of turning around a bit in front of a mirror to inject in the upper glutes close to the hip. Some have their partners or roommates inject them. Some others go through the trouble of visiting their doctor's nurse to inject. I think independence is important, so learn whatever works for you so that you do not need anyone else to do it for you.

For an update on injection techniques, please visit my web site TestosteroneWisdom.com for videos.

A note about subcutaneous versus intramuscular testosterone injections:

Dr. M.B. Greenspan and his team from McMaster University in Hamilton, Canada performed a pilot study in September 2005 of 10 men to assess the testosterone blood levels achieved by subcutaneous injections (SC) of testosterone compared to intramuscular injections. Every patient had been stable on testosterone enanthate (TE) at a dose of 200 mg intramuscularly (IM) for 1 year. Patients were instructed to self-inject with testosterone enanthate at 100 mg subcutaneously into the anterior abdomen once weekly. Some patients were down-titrated to 50 mg based on their total testosterone (T) at 4 weeks. T levels were measured before and 24 hours after injection during weeks 1, 2, 3, and 4, and 96 hours after injection in week 6 and 8. They concluded that a once-week SC injection of 50–100 mg of TE appears to achieve sustainable and stable levels of physiological T. This technique offers fewer physician visits and the use of smaller quantity of medication, thus lower costs. However, the long term clinical and physiological effects of this therapy need further evaluation.

Dr. Eugene Shippen, author of the 10 year old book "The Testosterone Syndrome" apparently prefers the SC injection method of testosterone replacement therapy in cases where he otherwise might have tried pellets, creams or gels. He claims that, unlike intramuscular injection, subcutaneous injection of a small amount three times per week results in more stable T levels and low estrogen conversion. Shippen's protocol includes SC injections of depo-testosterone 200mg/ml, .35 ml every 3 days into abdominal fat. He splits the injections into two .18 ml injections which is .36 ml, and says this is because a tiny amount will leak out of the injection site.

Esters of testosterone are dissolved in sesame or grape seed oil, which is very viscous and hard to inject through a small insulin syringe. But apparently, it can be done. I have never tried this protocol.

Transdermal Systems

Transdermal gels (Androgel, Testim)
As shown in Figure 10, creams and gels may provide lower and more sustained concentrations of testosterone in the blood without the "yo-yo" effect that injections can cause. Testosterone gets absorbed through the skin in a once or twice daily use.

The best application areas for the gel include the stomach, shoulders, the inner thighs, and the pectorals. Be aware that some people complain about dark hair growth where the cream or gel is applied, especially if one site is used over and over again without rotation.

Mean Steady-State Testosterone Concentrations in Patients Receiving AndroGel®

Day 90

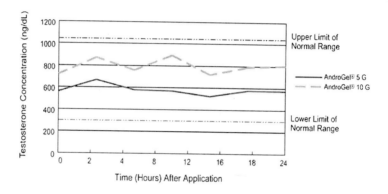

Figure 10. Testosterone blood levels are more stable on testosterone gels

As mentioned if you use testosterone this way, it can rub off onto a female partner or children when you hug them. So, it is important that this is kept in mind.

I think that its application on the back of the legs may help avoid this potential transfer of testosterone to other people. Most testosterone in gels and creams gets absorbed in the first one to two hours, but some residual testosterone may still be present after a few hours.

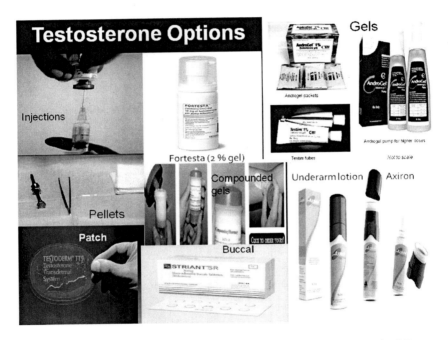

Figure 11. Commercially available testosterone products in the United States

Topical testosterone products represent approximately 65.6 percent of the total number of testosterone prescriptions dispensed between 2000 and November 2008, according to the FDA. Two prescription-based commercial testosterone gels are available in the United States: Androgel, approved by the FDA in February 2000, and Testim, approved in October 2002 (See Figure 11). Approximately 1.4 million prescriptions were dispensed for Androgel and 400,000 prescriptions were dispensed for Testim in 2008. The majority of prescriptions for Androgel are dispensed to adult males 50 to 59 years of age.

Both gels are colorless and evaporate quickly after being applied to the abdomen, shoulders, or arms. Androgel and Testim come in three dose levels (2.5 g, 5 g and 10 g with 1 percent testosterone each). Ten percent of the applied testosterone is absorbed into the blood stream through the skin. The usual starting dose is a packet of 5 g a day.

Androgel also comes in a pump that allows for higher dosing for those men who do not reach normal testosterone levels with the available gels. Each pump container is capable of dispensing 75 grams or 60 metered 1.25-gram doses. The starting dose of 5 grams a day requires four pump squirts. Many men require up to 10 grams per day to reach total testosterone blood levels above 500 ng/ml. This makes for eight squirts a day of Androgel. For some, that is a lot of volume to spread on the body. Luckily these gels dry up fast and leave little to no residue.

Auxilium, the maker of Testim, claims that their gel has a slightly better absorption rate than Androgel; however, many men do not like its slight soapy smell (Androgel has none).

Androgel and Testim are usually covered by insurance. Their monthly cost is around US$700 a month, with insurance co pays ranging from US$20 to US$50 a month. A patient assistance program has been set up by both companies to provide free drug to low-income patients with no insurance (read the resource section in this book for additional information).

At the time of writing this book, some companies were getting ready to manufacture generic testosterone gels which may provide a cheaper alternative.

Regardless of which gel you use, make sure your doctor re-checks your blood levels after two weeks to see whether you need to readjust the dose.

Figure 12 shows the areas where gels are usually applied. Testosterone gels should be applied to clean, dry skin. Do not apply to the testicular area since this has been shown to increase DHT conversion.

Application sites should be allowed to dry for a few minutes before dressing. Hands should be washed thoroughly with soap and water after application. In order to prevent transfer of testosterone to another person, clothing should be worn to cover the application sites. If a direct skin-to-skin contact with another person is anticipated, the application sites should be washed thoroughly with soap and water. Users should wait at least two hours after applying before showering or swimming; for optimal absorption, it may be best to wait five to six hours.

Men who may carry babies should be extra careful to avoid skin-to-skin contact after applying the gel since testosterone exposure in babies may have negative effects on the baby's growth. This fact was included in a recent label change for both Testim and Androgel described in the FDA web site: "Since the initial marketing approval of testosterone gel in 2000 to May 2009, FDA's Adverse Event Reporting System (AERS) received 20 reports (18 U.S. and 2 non-U.S.) describing adverse events in children who were exposed to testosterone gel that was used by another person (referred to as 'secondary exposure'). The adverse events reported in these children included one or more of the following signs or symptoms: enlargement of the penis or clitoris, premature development of pubic hair, advanced bone age, increased self-stimulation, libido, erections, and aggressive behavior. An increased testosterone level was reported in more than half of these cases. The children ranged in age from 9 months to 7 years. Three of the 20 cases are described in the medical literature." So, be careful not to come in contact with another person during first 4 hours of administration.

- **Abdomen**
- **Shoulders**
- **Upper arms**

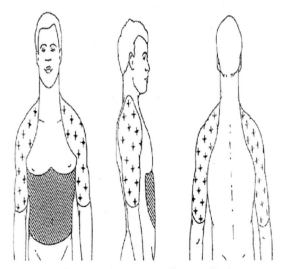

Figure 12. Body areas where gels are usually applied

Compounded creams and gels

Compounded creams and gels can be mixed by compounding pharmacies, and are similar in dosing, application, and precautions to what is described above for Androgel and Testim. There are various qualities of creams and gels made by compounding pharmacies around the United States, and some of the poorer quality products are gunky and flake off after they dry. Be sure to buy from a reputable pharmacy.

The best gels are clear and basically disappear shortly after application. Most men prefer alcohol-based gels, which absorb through the skin better than water-based gels. Creams should not be greasy and should resemble good moisturizing creams. Many compounding pharmacies make cheaper gels and creams with higher testosterone concentrations (2 to 10 percent) for men who do not respond to the commercially available 1 percent testosterone gel products (Testim or Androgel).

Some doctors do not feel comfortable prescribing gels from compounding pharmacies since they worry about quality control. There is also concern that higher concentration gels may induce more DHT conversion, which may cause more prostatic hyperplasia (inflammation) causing urinary flow restrictions especially in older men. Also, higher DHT can cause acne and hair loss.

There are many compounding pharmacies around the United States. I have used several compounding pharmacies in the past 15 years. For a list of compounding pharmacies, please visit TestosteroneWisdom.com

You can also Google the key words: "compounding pharmacy" and your zip code to find compounding pharmacies close to you. Compounding pharmacies ship across state lines, so it is not imperative that you have one in your area. They do not typically take insurance, so you have to request reimbursement from your insurance company. Your doctor has to be willing to call or fax a prescription to the pharmacy for you to order any testosterone products. The compounding pharmacy will need your credit card before shipping the product to you, so make sure you call them to set that up.

Most compounded testosterone gels of 1 to 10 percent concentrations can range between $17 and $70 a month so it's worth calling around for price comparisons. Your doctor may have an established relationship with a local compounding pharmacy, so be sure to ask. As mentioned before, some doctors have trust issues with compounding pharmacies' quality control and ask to see their certificates to prove that they have proper quality control standards.

There are two main advantages of using compounding pharmacies when getting a testosterone gel or cream. The first is cost: until a generic version of the gel is available, compounded gel will usually be the cheaper alternative. This is a non issue if you have an insurance policy that pays for the product and that it does not require you to pay high out of pocket co-pays when getting Androgel, Testim, Fortesta or Axiron.

The second is customization: your doctor can write a prescription of varying concentration for gels or creams. I have used gels containing 5 and 10 percent testosterone with great results. Of course the volume needed is lower when the concentration increases. Some researchers believe that higher concentration gels tend to increase DHT levels more strongly than the regular 1 percent gels. However many men need more than the usual amount of Testim or Androgel and do not want to smear their bodies with lots of gel, so 5 percent gels may be an option for them.

Most compounding pharmacies dispense the creams in "Topi-Click" (see Figure 13) that are more practical (typically) than the large pre-loaded syringes they are usually supplied in. The Topi-Click is more like a "deodorant stick" which can be more convenient and better looking than the bigger syringes.

Compounded Testosterone- TopiClick Applicator

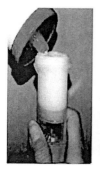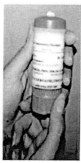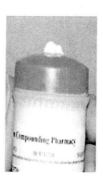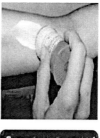

Figure 13. TopiClick Applicator for a compounded testosterone cream

PERSONAL COMMENT: I tried both Androgel and Testim for a few weeks. Both were effective but I admit to having a little sticker shock ($260 to $600 per month depending on dose, if not paid by insurance). Testim had a soapy smell that I didn't particularly like, but some women gave me compliments on my "cologne." I did like the large pump dispenser for Androgel since I could adjust the dosage if needed (I needed 10 grams of gel a day. Most doctors start you at 5 grams per day). I am currently using a testosterone gel/cream formulation with 5 percent testosterone. The prescription is written like this: *Testosterone gel/cream 5 percent 30 mL in Topi-Click, 1 mL a day.* I find the Topi-Click container to be a very easy way to administer the daily dose. You can also order the gel in a large graduated plastic syringe if you want to precise on your dose.

Transdermal patches

Another option for testosterone replacement therapy is a testosterone patch such as Testoderm or Androderm. For many men two 5-mg patches will bring them into the effective mid-range (500 ng/dL and above) of the testosterone blood test. The most frequent complaint with the patch is skin irritation at the application site. Some men do not like the potential of an unwanted "disclosure" since the patch can be visible to anyone who may see you without clothes. You also run the risk of having the patch fall off after sweating or bathing.

Androderm

Androderm comes in two doses: A 2.5 mg/patch and a 5.0 mg/patch. The actual amount of testosterone in the 2.5 mg patch is really 12.2 mg, while in the 5.0 mg patch it is 24.3 mg. Similar to what happens with the gel, much of the testosterone in the patch will not be absorbed into your system. So the aim of the 2.5 mg patch is to get 2.5 mg of testosterone successfully into the blood stream each day. It is possible to absorb slightly more or slightly less than the 2.5 mg patch's ideal dosage (this applies to the 5.0 mg patch as well). Most men need not one but two patches of 5 mg each to attain total testosterone blood levels above 500 ng/dL.

Androderm patches are usually applied on the back, abdomen, thighs, or upper arms. Because the active area of the patch is covered, you can enjoy some worry-free skin contact with your partner. As with any form of testosterone, your blood level will need to be checked by your doctor to readjust your dosage. Since dosages vary between 2.5 and 10 mg daily, this may require one or more patches.

It seems from the data that Androderm does not raise DHT or estrogen levels too much, so this may be an advantage for this option.

PERSONAL COMMENT: I have used Androderm and I have to say that I was not very fond of this product. I felt kind of exposed when I was naked, I didn't want to have to talk about testosterone replacement therapy just when things were getting interesting. Some countries and public clinics

provide only Androderm as the only option for TRT; it is a good option I
would not discourage anyone from using it.

Testoderm TTS

Testoderm was first introduced as a patch that you would have to apply to
the scrotum (testicular sack) after shaving it. For obvious reasons, it was
not very practical and discreet (imagine explaining to any sexual partners
what that patch is doing there and that you are not injured as it may seem!).
It also showed large increases in DHT since the scrotum tissue seems to
facilitate the conversion of testosterone into DHT. For this reason a new
non-scrotal patch was developed. Testoderm TTS patches are available in
two doses: 4.0 and 6.0 mg/patch. As with Androderm, the actual amount of
testosterone in these patches is greater than the listed dose because much
of the testosterone will not be absorbed.

Testoderm TTS patches are usually applied on the back, abdomen,
thighs, or upper arms. Since the patch is covered (like in the case of
Androderm) you don't have to worry about transferring the testosterone
through skin contact with a partner. Dosages will vary between 4.0 and 12
mg daily requiring one or more patches. Again, after a starting dose, your
testosterone level will need to be re-checked by your doctor a month after
to determine the right dose for you.

Anecdotally Testoderm TTS seems to increase DHT levels more than
most other options in the market, although a study showed constant
testosterone/DHT ratios, meaning that both values increased in the same
proportion.

Testosterone Pellets (Testopel or compounded pellets)

One other option for testosterone replacement therapy is the use pellets
inserted under the skin. These are small, sterile cylinders about the size
of a grain of rice that are produced by compressing medicated powders.
A doctor implants these pellets underneath the skin in the upper buttock
area by the hip. They can be used whenever a prolonged continuous
absorption of hormones is desired. Men who have problems remembering
daily applications, who are afraid of needles, or that travel a lot, may find
this option a very practical one.

Men receiving the pellet implants enjoy the convenience of not having
to worry about daily dosing normally or weekly injections associated with
other delivery systems. Testosterone implants have been around for many
years, but many doctors shy away from for several reasons:

•   Doctors need special training to learn the insertion technique;

- it is difficult to determine the optimal initial number of pellets, and is inconvenient to insert addition pellets if needed;
- the risks of infections in the insertion site.
- some users have reported problems with the pellets working their way out from under the skin (called extrusion).

Doctors can charge for the pellets (sold only to doctors), for the procedure, and all blood tests required, so pellets can be a good source of income for them.

The Testopel pellet—the only one approved by the FDA—contains 75 mg of testosterone. Testopel® Pellets (testosterone) are cylindrically shaped pellets 3.2mm (1/8 inch) in diameter and approximately 8-9mm in length. Each sterile pellet weighs approximately 77mg (75mg testosterone) and is ready for implantation. Depending on your body weight and metabolism, and pellet dose, 6–14 pellets are inserted in one procedure. The insertion of the pellets is quick and usually done using a local anesthetic. Pellets typically last for 3 to 4 months. Most patients return to work the day of or the day after implantation, but are advised to avoid bending or vigorous physical activity during this time.

Testopel's package insert says that the number of pellets to be implanted depends upon the minimal daily requirements of testosterone propionate determined by a gradual reduction of the amount administered parenterally. The usual dosage is as follows: implant two 75 mg pellets for each 25 mg testosterone propionate required weekly. Thus when a patient requires injections containing 100 mg per week, it is usually necessary to implant 600 mg of the pellet (8 pellets, each containing 75 mg).

Pellet implantation is much less flexible for dosage adjustment than is oral administration of or intramuscular injections of oil based esters. Therefore, great care should be used when estimating the amount of testosterone needed.

In the face of complications where the effects of testosterone should be discontinued, the pellets would have to be removed.

In addition, there are times when the pellets may slough out (extrusion). This accident is usually linked to superficial implantation or neglect in regard to aseptic precautions.

Some compounding pharmacies can also make testosterone pellets, though it is difficult to determine how effective they are. Compounded pellets can vary from 75 mg to 200 mg a pellet. Compounded pellets have been used for years for the treatment of low testosterone in women.

Medicaid reimburses $67.50 per pellet, and a 200-pound man usually needs 8-12 pellets to reach adequate blood levels, even though Testopel's package insert recommends 6 pellets. I have talked to some men that did not have insurance and both paid around $1,000 as a total cost for the pellets and doctor's fees. If this therapy is effective for four months, then the cost amounts to $250 a month. Several insurance companies do not reimburse for the pellets, but many are starting to do so. Medicare pays for them. But you will have to find a physician who has been trained on subcutaneous implantation of the pellets.

There is very little data on DHT or estrogen conversion of pellets, but it is speculated that they tend to have the fewest problems in that area for men.

Pellets are definitely an option to consider if you cannot adhere to daily gels or weekly injections. Some doctors are better than others at inserting them and at getting insurance to pay for this option. Make sure you ask the doctor how long he/she has been inserting pellets and what is his/her infection/extrusion rate.

PERSONAL COMMENT: I have used Testopel with great results. Twelve pellets were inserted under the skin of my upper buttocks area. My total testosterone went up from 350 NG/dL to 650 ng/dL and it stayed around 500 ng/dL for three and half months. It was so great not having to worry about remembering to inject every week or apply gel every day. The tiny pellets were not noticeable to the naked eye after the procedure and disappeared after four months. I want to send a big "thank you" to Dr. Richard Cavender in Ohio who did a great job inserting my pellets quickly and painlessly (www.nahealthassoc.com). He has a comprehensive wellness clinic with fancy computerized exercise equipment, nutritionists, and a whole gamut of wellness services. Definitely ahead of his time! I understand that he trains physicians on proper pellet insertion techniques. If my insurance paid for this option and I found a good doctor in Houston who would administer this option, I would probably use it as my first option since I have a busy life style and love not having to worry about weekly injections or daily gels.

Sublingual/buccal testosterone

The sublingual and buccal testosterone forms work by placing either a dissolving tablet under your tongue (sublingual) or a tablet against the surface of the gums (buccal). It is different from an oral delivery in that very little of the substance is swallowed, avoiding potential liver toxicity.

Sublingual

Sublingual testosterone can be obtained through compounding pharmacies as flavored, dissolvable tablets.

Usually 15 mg twice a day will bring total testosterone levels to over 500 ng/dL. Some men may need only once a day dosing. It is still good to check your testosterone blood levels two weeks after daily use to see whether the dose is right for you. It is claimed that no liver toxicities are associated with this option. Some men report a short-term boost in testosterone that may help with arousal right before sex.

PERSONAL COMMENT: I have tried some compounding pharmacies' mint-tasting products. I experienced no increase in my liver enzymes. However, it's twice a day application was not practical for my busy lifestyle.

Buccal

In 2003, the FDA approved Striant, a sustained-release buccal testosterone tablet. It is placed in the small depression in the mouth where the gum meets the upper lip, above the front teeth. Once applied, the tablet softens and delivers testosterone through the buccal mucosa, or gums. It is then absorbed directly into the blood stream, bypassing the liver and the rest of the gastrointestinal system. The recommended dosage for Striant is to replace the tablet about every 12 hours, though a different dosing schedule or number of tablets might be required depending on the total testosterone levels of the patient. Some men complain that the tablets fall off a few hours after application.

Some patients find this treatment too cumbersome. Others are concerned about the system shifting out of place or transferring testosterone to sexual partners via the saliva. Others may object to twice-daily dosing and would just as soon use daily gels. A bitter taste and gum inflammation can occur but usually resolves after the first week.

The average wholesale price of a 30-day supply of 30 mg buccal tablets for twice-daily dosing is US$190.30, or approximately US$6.34 a day.

This option has not really caught on, probably for obvious reasons.

PERSONAL COMMENT: I have not tried this option. No particular reason; I guess I was too busy trying other options and the thought of having something stuck to my gums was not really appealing. And the risk of transferring testosterone to someone you kiss is definitely there.

Human Chorionic Gonadotropin

Human chorionic gonadotropin (HCG) (not to be confused with human growth hormone, or HGH) is a glycoprotein hormone that mimics LH (luteinizing hormone), produced in pregnancy by the developing embryo soon after conception, and later by part of the placenta. Its role is to prevent the disintegration of the corpus luteum of the ovary and to maintain the progesterone production critical for pregnancy in women. It supports the normal development of an egg in a woman's ovary, and stimulates the release of the egg during ovulation. HCG is used to cause ovulation and to treat infertility in women.

You're probably asking yourself why you should care about this. But in men, HCG is also used in young boys when their testicles have not dropped down into the scrotum normally. Additionally, HCG is used to increase testicular size after long-term testosterone or anabolic steroid use.

As mentioned at the beginning of the book, testosterone replacement therapy triggers the hypothalamus to shut down its production of GnRH (gonadotropin releasing hormone). Without GnRH, the pituitary gland stops releasing LH. Without LH the testes (testicles or gonads) shut down their production of testosterone. For males HCG closely resembles LH. If the testicles have shrunken after long-term testosterone use, they will likely begin to enlarge and start their testosterone production shortly after HCG therapy is instituted. HCG jump-starts your testes to produce testosterone and to increase their size.

HCG can be extracted from pregnant women's urine or through genetic modification. The product is available by prescription under the brand names Pregnyl, Follutein, Profasi, and Novarel. Novire is another brand but it is a product of recombinant DNA. Compounding pharmacies can also make HCG by prescription in different vial sizes. Brand names of HCG in regular pharmacies cost over $100 per 10,000 IUs. The same amount of IUs cost around $50 in compounding pharmacies. Many insurance policies do not pay for HCG since they consider its use for testicular atrophy while on TRT an off label use. So, most men using it pay for it themselves and get it from compounding pharmacies that sell it a lot cheaper.

HCG is dispensed as a powder contained in vials of 3,500 IUs, 5, 000 IUs or 10, 000 IUs. You can call compounding pharmacies and have them make vials for you with different IU amounts, though. These are usually accompanied by another vial of 1 mL (or cc) of bacteriostatic water to

What is an IU? When measuring testosterone we spoke in weights of grams and milligrams. HCG is measured not by weight but in IU's, or international units. IU is not about weight but refers to the amount of a substance that produces a particular biologic effect that has been agreed upon as in international standard. The IU from one substance to the next does not mean they have equivalent weights (for example, 1, 000 IU of vitamin C might have a different weight than 1,000 IU of vitamin A). Again, IU is not a weight.

reconstitute the powder into a liquid solution. Bacteriostatic water (water with a preservative that is provided with the prescription) is mixed in with the powder to reconstitute, or dissolve, it before injection. This type of water can preserve the solution for up to 6 weeks when refrigerated. Some patients do not use the 1 mL water vials that come with the commercially (non compounded) available product and instead get their doctors to prescribe 30 cc bottles of bacteriostatic water so that they can dilute the HCG down to a more workable concentration that is more practical for men using lower doses of HCG weekly.

HCG is given as an injection under the skin or intramuscularly (there is still debate on which method is best). The number of IUs per injection will depend on how much bacteriostatic water you add to the dry powder vial. If you add 1 mL to a 5,000 IU powder vial, then you will have 5,000 IUs per mL, so 0.1 mL would be 500 IUs. If you add 2 mL to the 5,000 IU dry powder vial, then you will have 2,500 IUs/mL; 0.1 ml (or cc) in an insulin syringe will equal 250 IUs. If you need to inject 500 IUs, then you inject 0.2 ccs of this mixture. Table 3 provides dilution volumes at different HCG powder/water proportions.

Ultra-fine needle insulin syringes are used to inject HCG under the skin, making this very easy to take even for the needle-phobic. Typical sizes are:

- 1 ml, 12.7 mm long, 30 gauge and
- 0.5 ml, 8 mm, 31 gauge syringes.

Table 3. HCG Dilution Table

IUs of dry powder HCG	Amount of bacteriostatic water mixed in (cc)	Injection volume for 250 IU (cc)	Injection Volume for 500IU (cc)	Injection volume for 1000 IU (cc)
5,000	5	0.25	0.5	1
5,000	10	0.5	1	2
10,000	5	0.13	0.25	0.5
10,000	10	0.25	0.5	1

Syringes require a separate prescription. Some compounding pharmacies will automatically include them with the shipment, but do not forget to ask them. Never use the syringe that you used for injecting the bacteriostatic water into the powder for injecting yourself; the needle will be dull (I usually use a regular 23 gauge, 1 inch, 3 ml syringe to load up the water). Remember that you also need alcohol pads to clean the injection area and the tip of the vial. Typical injection sites are the abdominal area close to the navel or in the pubic fat pad. Pinch a little of fat on your abdominals and inject into that pinched area, then massage with an alcohol pad. Discard syringes into the sharps container that can be provided by your pharmacy.

As I mentioned before, compounded HCG is a lot cheaper than the commercially available pharmaceutical products. Sometimes it is difficult to find commercially available HCG in regular pharmacies.

A review of the literature reveals a wide range of doses of HCG used and that there is very little agreement among physicians. For male infertility, doses range from 1250 IU three times weekly to 3000 IU twice weekly (these studies did not include men on testosterone replacement).

How long does the boost in testosterone last after an injection of HCG? A study looked into that and also tried to determine if high doses would be more effective at sustaining that boost. The profiles of plasma testosterone and HCG in normal adult men were studied after the administration of 6000 IU HCG under two different protocols. In the first protocol, seven subjects received a single intramuscular injection. Plasma testosterone increased sharply (1.6 ± 0.1-fold) within 4 hours. Then testosterone decreased slightly and remained at a plateau level for at least 24 hours. A delayed peak of testosterone (2.4 ± 0.3-fold) was seen between 72–96 hours. Thereafter, testosterone declined and reached the initial levels at 144 hours. In the second protocol, six subjects received two intravenous (IV) injections of HCG (5-8 times the dose given by injection to the first group) at 24-hour intervals. The initial increment of plasma testosterone after the first injection was similar to that seen in the first protocol despite the fact that plasma HCG levels were 5–8 times higher in this case. At 24 hours, testosterone levels were again lower than those observed at 2–4 hours and a second IV injection of HCG did not induce a significant increase. The delayed peak of plasma testosterone (2.2 ± 0.2-fold of control) was seen about 24 hour later than that in the first protocol. So, this study shows that more is not better when dosing HCG. In fact, high doses may desensitize Leydig cells in the testicles. It also showed that testosterone blood levels peak not once but twice after HCG injections. I wish they had studied a lower dose than 6000 IU since very few physicians prescribe this high dose.

HCG may not only boost testosterone but also increase the number of Leydig cells in the testicles. It is well known that Leydig cell clusters in adult testes enlarge considerably under treatment with HCG. However, it has been uncertain in the past whether this expansion involves an increase in the number of Leydig cells or merely an enlargement of the individual cells. A study was performed in which adult male Sprague-Dawley rats were injected subcutaneously daily with 100 IU HCG for up to 5 weeks. The volume of Leydig cell clusters increased by a factor of 4.7 during the 5 weeks of HCG treatment. The number of Leydig cells (initially averaging 18.6 x 106/cm3 testis) increased to 3 times the control value by 5 weeks of treatment ($P<0.001$), while the average volume of individual Leydig cells (initially ~2200 μm3) enlarged only 1.6 times. They concluded that chronic treatment with HCG increases the number of Leydig cells in the testes of adult rats. We do not know if these results can be extrapolated to men.

Currently there are no HCG guidelines for men who need to be on testosterone replacement therapy and want to maintain normal testicular size. A study that used 200 mg per week of testosterone enanthate injections with HCG at doses of 125, 250, or 500 IU every other day in healthy younger men showed that the 250 IU dose every other day preserved normal testicular function (no testicular size measurements were taken, however). Whether this dose is effective in older men is yet to be proven. Also, there are no long-term studies using HCG for more than 2 years.

Due to its effect on testosterone, HCG use can also increase estradiol and DHT, although I have not seen data that shows if this increase is proportional to the dose used.

So, the best dose of HCG to sustain normal testicular function while keeping estradiol and DHT conversion to a minimum has not been established (I will explain why these two metabolites are important in TRT management).

Some doctors are recommending using 200–500 IUs twice a week for men who are concerned about testicular size or who want to preserve fertility while on testosterone replacement. Higher doses, such as 1,000–5,000 IUs twice a week, have been used but I believe that these higher doses could cause more estrogen and DHT-related side effects, and possibly desensitize the testicles for HCG in the long term. Some doctors check estradiol levels a month after this protocol is started to determine whether the use of the estrogen receptor modulators tamoxifen (brand name: Nolvadex) or anaztrozole (brand name: Arimidex), is needed to counteract any increases in estradiol levels. High estradiol can cause breast enlargement and water retention in men but it is important at the right blood levels to maintain bone and brain health (refer to the Gynecomastia section for more on this subject).

Shippen's Chorionic Gonadotrophin Stimulation Test (for males under 75 years of age)

Even though there seems not be an accepted and clinically proven protocol to dose HCG, Dr. Eugene Shippen (author of the book "The Testosterone Syndrome"), has developed his own after his own experiences. Most doctors do not follow this protocol but I am showing it here since I get a lot of questions about it. I have never used this protocol myself since I have been on testosterone replacement for over 15 years.

Dr. Shippen has found that a typical treatment course for three weeks is best for determining those individuals who will respond well to HCG treatment. It is administered daily by injection 500 units subcutaneously, Monday through Friday for three weeks. The patient is taught to self administer with 50 Unit insulin syringes with 30 gauge needles in anterior thigh, seated with both hands free to perform the injection. Testosterone, total and free, plus E2 (estradiol) are measured before starting the protocol and on the third Saturday after 3 weeks of stimulation (he claims that salivary testing may be more accurate for adjusting doses). Studies have shown that subcutaneous injections are equal in efficacy to intramuscular administration.

By measuring the effect on his HCG protocol on total testosterone, he identifies candidates that require testosterone replacement versus those who just require having their testicles "awaken" with HCG to produce normal testosterone. I am yet to see any data that substantiates his approach, however.

Here is how he determines leydig (testicular) cell function:

1. If the HCG protocol causes less than a 20% rise in total testosterone he suggests poor testicular reserve of leydig cell function (primary hypogonadism or eugonadotrophic hypogonadism indicating combined central and peripheral factors).

2. 20-50% increase in total testosterone indicates adequate reserve but slightly depressed response, mostly central inhibition but possibly decreased testicular response as well.

3. More than 50% increase in total testosterone suggests primarily centrally mediated depression of testicular function.

He then offers these options for treatment for patients depending on the response to HCG and patient determined choices.

1. If there is an inadequate response (< 20%), then replacement with testosterone will be indicated.

2. The area in between 20-50% will usually require HCG boosting for a period of time, plus natural boosting or "partial" replacement options.

    I am yet to see what he means with natural boosting!

    Dr. Shippen believes that full replacement with testosterone is always the last option in borderline cases since improvement over time may frequently occur as the testicles' leydig cell regeneration may actually happen. He claims that much of this is age dependent. Up to age 60, boosting is almost always successful. In the age range 60-75 is variable, but will usually be clear by the results of the stimulation test. Also, disease related depression of testosterone output might be reversible with adequate treatment of the underlying process (depression, obesity, alcohol, deficiency, etc.) He claims that this positive effect will not occur if suppressive therapy is instituted in the form of full testosterone replacement.

3. If there is an adequate response of more than 50% rise in testosterone, there is very good leydig cell reserve. HCG therapy will probably be successful in restoring full testosterone output without replacement, a better option over the long term and a more natural restoration of biologic fluctuations for optimal response. But I am yet to see any data on long term use of HCG used in this approach! (I invite researchers to do such studies)

4. Chorionic HCG can be self-administered and adjusted according to

response. In younger, high output responders (T > 1100ng/dl), HCG can be given every third or fourth day. This also minimizes estrogen conversion. In lower level responders (600-800ng/dl), or those with a higher estradiol output associated with full dose HCG, 300-500 units can be given Mon-Wed-Fri. At times, sluggish responders may require a higher dose to achieve full testosterone response.

Dr. Shippen believes in checking salivary levels of free testosterone on the day of the next injection, but before the next injection to determine effectiveness and to adjust the dose accordingly. He claims that later as leydig cell restoration occurs, a reduction in dose or frequency of administration may be later needed.

5. He recommends to monitor both testosterone and estradiol levels to assess response to treatment after 2 - 3 weeks after change in dose of HCG as well as periodic intervals during chronic administration. He claims that salivary testing will better reflect the true free levels of both estrogens and testosterone. (Pharmasan.com and others) Most insurance companies do not pay for salivary testing. Blood testing is the standard way to test for testosterone and estradiol.

6. Except for reports of antibodies developing against HCG (he mentions that he has never seen this problem), the claims that there are no adverse effects of chronic HCG administration.

Dr. Shippen's book was published in the late 90's. I know of no physician that uses his protocol. I have no opinion on its validity. The idea that testicular function can be improved with cycles of HCG in men with low testosterone caused by sluggish yet functioning leydig cells is an interesting concept that needs to be studied. I guess that since this protocol requires very close monitoring, many doctors have avoided using it. The off label nature of the protocol's use of HCG can also make it expensive for patients who will have to pay cash for its use and monitoring.

A very well known doctor in the field of testosterone replacement, Dr. John Crisler (www.allthingsmale.com), recommends 250IU of HCG twice per week for all TRT patients, taken the day of, along with the day before, the weekly testosterone cypionate injection. After looking at countless lab printouts, listening to subjective reports from patients, and learning more about HCG, he reports to be shifting that regimen forward one day. In other words, his patients who inject testosterone cypionate now take their HCG at 250IU two days before, as well as the day immediately previous to, their weekly intramuscular shot. All administer their HCG subcutaneously, and dosage may be adjusted as necessary (he reports that rarely more than 350 IU twice weekly dose is required).

For men using testosterone gels, the same dose every third day has anecdotally helps to preserve testicular size (the dose of the gel has to be adjusted after a month of HCG to compensate for the increased testosterone caused by HCG).

Some doctors believe that stopping TRT for a few weeks in which only 1000- 2000 IU HCG weekly is used provides a good way to stimulate testicular function without having to use HCG continuously. I have not seen any data to support this approach. Others believe that cycling HCG on and off while maintaining TRT may prevent any desentization of testicular Leydig cells to HCG. Again, no data or reports have been published on this approach.

Some men have asked me why we cannot use HCG solely to make our own testicles produce testosterone without the use of TRT along with it. According to Dr. Crisler, using HCG as sole testosterone replacement option does not bring the same subjective benefit on sexual function as pure testosterone delivery systems do—even when similar serum androgen levels are produced from comparable baseline values. However, supplementing the more "traditional" transdermal, or injected options, testosterone with the correct doses of HCG stabilizes blood levels, prevents testicular atrophy, helps rebalance expression of other hormones, and brings reports of greatly increased sense of well-being and libido. But in excess, HCG can cause acne, water retention, moodiness, and gynecomastia (breast enlargement in men).

Many men have complained that their doctors do not know about HCG and how to use it (I do not blame doctors for being confused!). Some spend a lot of time trying to find doctors to feel comfortable prescribing it. One good way to find out what doctor in your area may be currently prescribing it is to call your local compounding pharmacies to ask them what doctors call them for their patients' prescriptions.

If you decide (with the agreement of your doctor) that you want to use HCG with your TRT regimen at 500 IU per week, then you will need 2000 IU per month. I personally do not like to have diluted HCG sitting in my fridge for over six weeks (HCG may degrade with time after mixed in with bacteriostatic water even when refrigerated). So, a 3000 or 35000 IU vial should suffice for 6 weeks. Your doctor can call in the following prescription to a compounding pharmacy:

Human Chorionic Gonadotropin, 3500 IU vial, #1, 3 refills, as directed

Every 5 weeks, remember to call the compounding pharmacy to get the next shipment of HCG so that you do not run out.

After reading this section, you probably agree with me that using HCG requires a lot of discipline since you have to remember to inject it weekly in addition to your weekly or bi-weekly testosterone injection. But I know of many men who have that type of commitment since they do not want testicular size reduction. And many of us may just be fine with our reduced testicular size as long as testosterone is actually doing its job in improving our sex drive. And some lucky men do not get testicular atrophy at all on testosterone (those with large testicles to start with usually do not seem to complain about shrinkage as much as men starting with smaller testicular size before TRT). So it is a personal decision at the end!

As you will read in the section "HPGA dysfunction" HCG is also used in a protocol in combination with clomid and tamoxifen to attempt to bring the body's own testosterone production back to normal when someone needs to stop testosterone or anabolic steroids after long-term use. This protocol only works for those who started testosterone or anabolic steroids at normal baseline testosterone levels (bodybuilders and athletes) and it is not intended to work in those of us who had testosterone deficiency (hypogonadism) to start with.

As you can tell, there is no agreement on the correct dose and frequency of HCG. I really hope that researchers in the endocrine field compare different protocols in a controlled manner so that we can settle this issue once and for all. I encourage pharmaceutical companies to seek approval for using HCG for prevention of testicular atrophy in men using TRT. This new indication can prove to be lucrative as the TRT market grows over 2 billion dollars a year in the United States as more men become aware of hypogonadism treatment options.

PERSONAL COMMENT: I have used HCG to reverse testicular shrinkage and it works extremely well not only for that purpose but also for boosting sexy drive. I do have to remind myself that as soon as I stop using it, testicular atrophy will recur. I have recently started using it in small doses (250 IU twice a week subcutaneously) which seems to be a good maintenance regimen for me. I get my HCG from compounding pharmacies at $70 per 10,000 IUs since the pharmaceutical commercial products are too expensive and rarely paid by insurance for testicular atrophy. I remind men that HCG can increase your estradiol and DHT blood levels, so it is important to have your doctor retest you for both of these values after you start. Lowering testosterone dosage may be required when using HCG along side with TRT since HCG can have an additive effect on testosterone blood levels. But we need so much more data on HCG to stop making assumptions and using protocols that are endorsed by anecdotal information.

Clomid (Clomiphene Citrate)

The following section could also be applied if talking about Arimidex (anastrazole) and letrozole (Femara), two non steroidal aromatase inhibitors that may decrease estradiol and increase testosterone.

While testosterone replacement is the most commonly used treatment for testosterone deficiency, it can lead to decreased sperm count and possible infertility (more on this later). It may be a less effective physiologic therapy for patients with secondary hypogonadism due to pituitary dysfunction. Clomiphene citrate (brand name Clomid) is believed by some to allow for restoration of testicular function by restoring physiologic pituitary function in some men with hypogonadism (this statement has not been proven in clinical studies). Clomiphene citrate increases LH and testosterone. It does not appear to down regulate testicular Leydig cell activity, because it blocks testicular estrogen receptors.

Clomiphene citrate is a selective estrogen receptor (ER) modulator approved in 1967 for the treatment of female infertility. It should be noted that most of the data for clomiphene were obtained through studies conducted in women, and good studies with its use in men have yet to be conducted (there is a company setting up research studies to explore the use of clomiphene in men with hypogonadism induced by long term anabolic steroid use). Clomiphene citrate's mechanism of action is primarily as an "antiestrogen." It occupies estrogen receptors and "deceives" the hypothalamus into sensing a low estrogen environment. This activity enhances the hypothalamus' release of GnRH, which impacts the HPGA by stimulating release of FSH and LH from the pituitary. Clomiphene citrate may provide an approach to hormone replacement that is more similar to the normal physiology of the HPGA compared with testosterone replacement therapy, and it may preserve fertility. However, several studies evaluating clomiphene citrate for the treatment of male infertility have produced mixed results. Further study will be needed to clarify the compound's potential utility in this indication.

But can clomiphene improve sexual function in men without the co-current use of testosterone? To answer this question, Dr. Guay and his team at the Center for Sexual Function in Peabody, Massachusetts, studied the effect of clomiphene citrate on primary hypogonadism (testicles themselves aren't producing enough testosterone) and erectile dysfunction in 272 men who have never used testosterone. Of these 272 trial participants, 228 completed a four-month regimen of clomiphene citrate dosed at 50 mg three times a week.

Mean age of these 173 men was 54.3 years. After four months of treatment, 75.1 percent of subjects reported improvement in erectile dysfunction including 38.7 percent who reported normal sexual function. The other 24.8 percent reported no change in erectile dysfunction. Serum LH and testosterone levels increased significantly compared with baseline values in all groups (responders, partial responders, and non-responders).

Importantly, clomiphene citrate did not result in supraphysiologic (higher than normal) levels of testosterone in this study, and testosterone levels were maintained within a normal range. Multivariate analysis revealed that age was the patient characteristic most predictive of positive or partial response to clomiphene citrate, with patients aged 55 years and younger more likely to respond compared with patients aged 56 years or older. Free testosterone blood levels were not reported, so it is difficult to attain why there was a difference in response in older men.

For dosing and a protocol that uses clomiphene, HCG and tamoxifen to help to normalize the HPGA after testosterone or anabolic use, please refer to the HPGA dysfunction section and in the Chapter 7 (interview with Dr. Michael Scally).

More studies are needed using clomiphene citrate alone or in combination with HCG and/or tamoxifen or anastrozole so that doctors feel more comfortable prescribing these compounds to help balance the HPGA.

Practical matters to keep in mind: Some men report experiencing mood changes and feel more emotional when using clomiphene citrate. I have not seen any data on Clomiphene's effects on estradiol levels, so it is unknown if this reported mood changes are due to higher estradiol. Clomiphene citrate can be quite expensive, although it can be found at lower prices at compounding pharmacies by prescription. Many doctors do not like to prescribe it due to the limited available data and the fact that it is not approved for men. Some doctors prescribe it off-label and patients pay for it out of their own pockets. It is not a controlled substance under the US Drug Enforcement Agency (DEA). Some men order it for personal use from websites of overseas companies at very low prices.

PERSONAL COMMENT: I have tried using clomiphene as a sole source of testosterone replacement. It did not work. My testosterone remained low and I experienced all symptoms of testosterone deficiency. I have talked to other men who have tried clomiphene with similar lack of efficacy. The discrepancy between my results with Dr. Guay's study (which enrolled hypogonadal men with no prior testosterone experience) may be explained by the fact that we had been on testosterone for years before starting clomiphene. No studies have looked into its use in men like me. This is one of the reasons that are simplistic to assume that a drug will work for anyone because studies have shown benefits in some patients. That is the main reason I wanted to try products before writing about them.

Newer Products:

Axiron, an underarm gel:

In an attempt to reduce the risk of transference of testosterone to others, a company called Acrux developed Axiron, a testosterone underarm product.

Axiron is the first testosterone topical solution approved for application via an armpit (underarm) applicator.

Axiron has been studied in 155 men in six countries and 26 sites. The data submission package for Axiron included findings from a Phase III multi-center, open label, 120-day clinical study which demonstrated that 84 percent of men who completed the study achieved average serum testosterone concentration within the normal range of 300-1050 ng/dL. Additionally, after 120 days of treatment, 75 percent of responding patients finished the study on the recommended starting dose of 60 mg.

The most common adverse reactions (incidence>4%) in this Phase III study were skin application site reactions, increased red blood cell count, headache, diarrhea, vomiting and an increase in blood level of Prostate Specific Antigen (a test used to screen for prostate cancer).

With this product men were permitted to use an underarm deodorant or antiperspirant during the trial. More than half of the men continued to apply an underarm deodorant or antiperspirant as part of their daily routine. An analysis of these subgroups showed that this had no impact on the efficacy of Axiron treatment.

Axiron comes in a pump. Your doctor should start you at an initial dose and then retest your testosterone two weeks to a month later to determine if dose readjustment is needed. The following dosing information is provided in the package insert:

Daily dose- Number of pump applications

30 mg (once daily). Swipe once on one underarm only (right OR left).

60 mg (once daily). Swipe once on the left AND once on the right underarm.

90 mg (once daily). Swipe once on the left AND once on the right underarm. Wait for AXIRON to dry. Then swipe again once on EITHER the right OR the left underarm.

120 mg (once daily). Swipe once on the left AND once on the right underarm. Wait for AXIRON to dry. Then apply once again on the left AND once again on the right underarm.

* Pumps = applications.

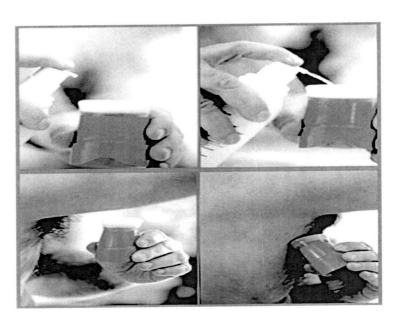

Figure 14. Axiron, an underarm testosterone gel

Fortesta, a 2 percent gel:

The same company that is hoping to launch Aveed (Nebido) in the United States, Endo Pharmaceuticals, received FDA approval in 2011 for Fortesta (testosterone) 2% Gel for men diagnosed with low testosterone. This gel contains more testosterone than Abbott's Androgel (which contains 1.62% testosterone).

Fortesta Gel is a clear, colorless, odorless gel that is gently applied with one finger to the front and inner thighs, and not the upper body. Fortesta gel comes in a metered-dose pump that delivers the correct dose per complete depression. Patients using Fortesta Gel should apply the product as directed. Safety and efficacy of Fortesta Gel in males less than 18 years old have not been established.

In a 90-day, multicenter, open-label, non-comparative, pivotal Phase III trial involving men with hypogonadism, 78 percent of patients using Fortesta gel had an average serum total testosterone concentration within the normal range at day 90. The most common side effect in this trial was application site reactions.

To avoid transferring testosterone to others who may come in contact with your skin, Endo says that you should apply Fortesta gel only to the front and inside area of your thighs that will be covered by clothing and to wash your hands right away with soap and water after applying it. After the gel has dried, cover the application area with clothing and keep the area covered until you have washed the application area well or have showered. If you expect another person to have skin-to-skin contact with your thighs, first wash the application area well with soap and water.

The company has a 30 day free coupon trial (with a prescription from your doctor). Go to Fortesta.com to download the coupon that you should take to your pharmacy along with your prescription.

Upcoming Products:

Nasobol, nasal spray:

A novel preparation of testosterone replacement in the form of a nasal gel (Nasobol) administered simultaneously to each nostril, has recently been subjected to clinical trials (phase II) in hypogonadal men.

Nasal applications lacks many of the different disadvantages of other products such as skin-to-skin transfer, stickiness, unpleasant smell (Testim), skin irritation (patches), elevated DHT (patches and oral), and injection pain and high T and DHT peaks (intramuscular injection). Instead, nasal application is simple and easy to use. Testosterone levels after nasal application follow the normal diurnal pattern of serum testosterone for the greater part of the day whereas virtually all other products give more or less "constant" steady state levels.

I have not seen side effect data on this product. It concerns me to be using a nasal spray that may affect the internal mucosa of the nose. I am looking forward to seeing data on sneezing, sinusitis, and sense of smell changes.

Libigel, the first gel for women:
Treatment with LibiGel in BioSante's Phase II clinical trial significantly increased satisfying sexual events in surgically menopausal women suffering from female sexual dysfunction (FSD).

FSD covers at least four different conditions: problems with desire, arousal, achieving orgasm, and genital pain. To establish a diagnosis of FSD, these syndromes must be associated with personal distress, as determined by the affected woman. A February 10, 1999 study published in the Journal of the American Medical Association, titled, "Sexual Dysfunction in the United States: Prevalence and Predictors," states that approximately 43% of postmenopausal women suffer from some form of FSD. There are no drugs in the United States approved for FSD indications.

The Phase II trial results showed LibiGel significantly increased the number of satisfying sexual events by 238% versus baseline (p<0.0001); this increase also was significant versus placebo (p<0.05). In this study the effective dose of LibiGel produced testosterone blood levels within the normal range for pre-menopausal women and had a safety profile similar to that observed in the placebo group. In addition, no serious adverse events and no discontinuations due to adverse events occurred in any subject receiving LibiGel. The Phase II clinical trial was a double-blind, placebo-controlled trial, conducted in the United States.

On January 24, 2008, the US FDA notified BioSante that it had completed and reached agreement with BioSante on a Special Protocol Assessment (SPA) for BioSante's Phase III safety and efficacy clinical trials of LibiGel in the treatment of hypoactive sexual desire syndrome (HSDD).

Both Phase III safety and efficacy trials are underway and are double-blind, placebo-controlled trials that have enrolled approximately 500 surgically menopausal women each for six-months of treatment.

There are questions about safety of testosterone therapy in women, even though there are no data to indicate that low dose testosterone causes any serious adverse events in women. Therefore, in addition to the two Phase III safety and efficacy trials described above, BioSante is conducting one Phase III cardiovascular safety study of LibiGel. The safety study is a randomized, double-blind, placebo-controlled, multi-center, cardiovascular events driven study of between 2,400 and 3,100 women exposed to LibiGel or placebo for 12 months. At the end of 12 months BioSante intends to submit a LibiGel new drug application (NDA) for review and possible approval by FDA. BioSante will continue to follow the women enrolled in the safety study for an additional four years after the NDA submission and possible approval of LibiGel.

Intrinsa, a testosterone patch for women:
Intrinsa is a testosterone patch by Procter & Gamble (P&G) designed to treat Female Sexual Dysfunction (FSD).

The patch aims to increase libido in women. Doctors have used a range of other treatments for women, including various hormones, antidepressants, and male impotence drugs like Viagra, Levitra, and Cialis. According to a P&G survey on female health 30 million women are naturally menopausal, 3 million are distressed by their lack of sexual desire, and 20% of 25 million women who are surgically menopausal are distressed.

Intrinsa works by releasing testosterone through the skin into the bloodstream. In women, testosterone is naturally produced by the ovaries and the adrenal gland. However, levels of the hormone decline with age, sometimes dramatically so after the menopause or after a hysterectomy. Testosterone therapy is systemic and needs to be applied over a period of weeks or months to have a noticeable effect.

The amount of testosterone in the patch, 300 μg/24hrs, is significantly lower than in testosterone patches for men. The patch is virtually transparent and about the size of an egg and is worn just below the navel and changed twice weekly.

In P&G's studies over six months of surgically menopausal women, those who received a placebo said satisfying sexual activity increased by an average of 19%, vs. a 73% increase for Intrinsa patch users.

The patch was granted a license from the European Medicines Agency. However, in December 2004 the United States the 14-member Food and Drug Administration (FDA) advisory committee, plus voting consultants, for Reproductive Health Drugs unanimously rejected Procter and Gamble's fast-track request for Intrinsa citing concerns about off-label use. In Canada, post-menopausal women have been able to obtain government-approved testosterone treatment since 2002.

It is not known if P&G will try to obtain approval of Intrinsa again in the United States, although I believe that if Libigel gets approved there is no reason for them not to do it. It amazes me that women in the United States have not been upset by the dismissal of sexual dysfunction in females by the approval process. I am glad to see this field moving along!

Selective Androgen Receptor Modulators

Oral selective androgen receptor modulators (SARMs) are investigational agents. Studied since 1998, they are still very much in the infancy of their development and marketing. SARMs may be able to provide the benefits of increased muscle mass and bone density, and fat loss that testosterone and other traditional anabolic/androgenic steroids provide but without the unwanted side effects (prostatic enlargement). SARMs are not intended to be a form of testosterone replacement therapy. So, why am I talking about them? Besides replacement therapy, testosterone and other anabolics can be useful in the treatment of certain aspects of disease. This is a topic close to my heart since this kind of medical use saved my life and that of many others. I spent years researching it to co-write the book "Built to Survive: A Comprehensive Guide to the Medical Use of Anabolic Therapies, Nutrition and Exercise for HIV+ Men and Women" (published in 1999 and then two more editions a few years later and available on amazon.com). Excuse me while I digress from the current topic.

Unintentional weight loss is common in a number of medical conditions (e.g., HIV/AIDS, burns, trauma, cancer, chronic obstructive pulmonary disease). The loss of too much weight, especially muscle mass, increases the risk of complications, including death. Dr. Donald Kotler from New York was able to plot body cell mass data versus mortality from different pathologies and found that once you lose 50% of your normal body cell mass, you die. So, there seems to be a minimum amount of lean tissue that the body needs to stay alive and functioning. Fat mass has not been correlated to increased survival, although losing fat has been proven to improve cardiovascular risks.

Cancer cachexia, or the unintentional loss of muscle mass and body weight, may lead to a loss of protein stores, severe weakness and fatigue, immobility and a loss of independence. It can impair the ability to tolerate and to respond to cancer treatments. An estimated 1.3 million cancer patients in the United States have cancer cachexia. Cancer-induced muscle wasting is thought to be responsible for greater than 20 percent of cancer deaths.

There are no drugs currently approved for the treatment of cancer cachexia. Physicians often prescribe different medications that have the side of effect of increased appetite in an attempt to fight weight loss. Megace, a progesterone-based appetite stimulant, is commonly used to increase

#200   10-17-2014 3:59PM
Item(s) checked out to SHOWALTER, DEANNE

TITLE: Testosterone: a man's guide : pra
BARCODE: 32233003339362
DUE DATE: 11-07-14

$1/day late fee for DVDs & videogames
$1 de multa por dia cada DVD/juego tarde

weight. Unfortunately most of this weight consists of fat (lean body mass, not fat gain, has been correlated to increased survival.) Megace also increases the chances for blood clots, high blood sugar and bone death.

Anabolics like nandrolone undecanoate and oxandrolone have been prescribed by progressive physicians to treat wasting in patients with non-androgen dependent cancers (colon, throat, lung, stomach, etc.) and HIV associated wasting. Androgens are contraindicated for people with prostate and breast cancer, as they can worsen these types of cancers. Anabolics are usually prescribed along with testosterone replacement even if the patient starting them for wasting syndrome has normal testosterone levels. Anabolics have the same inhibiting effect as testosterone on the HPGA and they decrease testosterone blood levels if no testosterone is used in combination with them. Many doctors fail to remember this and treat patients who are wasting with anabolics alone, which results in loss of sexual function in patients using them for a few weeks. So, testosterone replacement is essential as an adjunctive therapy when prescribing oxandrolone or nandrolone to patients with HIV, cancer, or other debilitating wasting conditions.

Oxandrolone (brand name: Oxandrin), an oral anabolic agent, is FDA approved as "adjunctive therapy to promote weight gain after weight loss following extensive surgery, chronic infections, or severe trauma, and in some patients who without definite pathophysiologic reasons fail to gain or to maintain normal weight, to offset the protein catabolism associated with prolonged administration of corticosteroids, and for the relief of bone pain frequently accompanying osteoporosis." (From the products package insert). Adjunctive means it is an additive or supportive therapy but it does not treat the *underlying* condition directly. In some patients and depending on the dose and duration, oxandrolone can increase liver enzymes and/or decrease high density cholesterol (HDL), the good cholesterol. Both side effects reverse when the drug is stopped. The usual dose for men is 20 mg/day (it can be used in women with wasting at 5-10 mg/day). As previously mentioned, testosterone is needed with it since it reduces testosterone and potentially sexual function after a few weeks in some patients. It is expensive at $1200 per month for 20 mg/day but insurance companies pay for it with some restrictions.

Nandrolone decanoate (brand name: Deca Durabolin), an injectable anabolic steroid, is the most studied anabolic agent for wasting syndrome. It requires a weekly injection of 200-400 mg plus testosterone replacement (100-200 mg testosterone cypionate a week or 5-10 grams of testosterone gel per day). Nandrolone is legally prescribed in an off-label manner to treat wasting syndrome since it is indicated for the management of the anemia of renal insufficiency and has been shown to increase hemoglobin and red cell mass. No liver toxicity has been reported in the many studies, but decreases in HDL and other side effects typical of testosterone have been observed in those using higher doses. Nandrolone is no longer available in regular pharmacies but it is available cheaply in compounding pharmacies by prescription (there is a list in the Appendix section). The average cost for 200 mg/week is $40 per month and it may produce the same effects on lean body mass than oxandrolone at 20 mg/day. Both nandrolone and oxandrolone can have the same side effects of testosterone (polycythemia and gynecomastia).

The only drug that is actually approved in the United States for HIV wasting syndrome that does not require an off label prescription is Serostim (human growth hormone made by Serono), although doctors prescribe oxandrolone and nandrolone a lot more due to cost and lower side effects. Depending on the dose used, Serostim can cost $3000 to $6000 per month. This product can cause joint aches, water retention, and irreversible diabetes. More details on treatment of wasting syndrome can be found in the previously mentioned book "Built to Survive" which I co-authored with Michael Mooney (the book is available on Amazon.com in a print or electronic version and has been translated into Spanish).

Low doses of growth hormone (growth hormone replacement therapy) are commonly prescribed in antiaging and men's clinics. It is a controversial topic that is beyond of the scope of this book. A lot of details are provided in 'Built to Survive."

So back to the SARMs:

SARMs are aimed to have the same benefits as anabolics but without the side effects.

Ostarine is an oral agent that has demonstrated the ability to increase lean body mass and improve muscle strength and performance in postmenopausal women, elderly men, and men and women with cancer cachexia. Ostarine is made by the company GTx's and has been studied in seven Phase I, Phase II, and Phase IIb clinical trials in 582 subjects.

It had no serious adverse events reported, although I am yet to see the data. Ostarine also exhibited no apparent change in measurements of serum prostatic specific antigen (PSA), sebum production (which causes acne), or decreases in blood levels of LH (which hints that it may not affect the HPGA at the doses tested). I have not seen LDL or HDL and hematocrit or hemoglobin data on this product to assess its effect on lipids and red blood cells, respectively. I am also curious about its effect on liver enzymes.

SARMs have anecdotally not helped increase sexual function, so they probably will not replace testosterone for treatment of hypogonadism. They also decrease the body's production of testosterone, just like anabolic steroids do. So, testosterone replacement will most probably be still required with their use for illness or aging associated loss of lean body mass. We await more data on these interesting compounds as they may have the same clinical benefits as anabolic steroids without the stigma and possibly without their side effects.

-4-

Monitoring Testosterone Replacement Therapy

Testosterone replacement therapy is not without side effects, although most are manageable and reversible after it is stopped. I've been taking testosterone replacement since 1993 and for the most part have had no side effects thanks to careful monitoring. It's critical that you are monitored for side effects in addition to your testosterone level. Some men may experience one or more side effects that sometimes go unnoticed until they become aware of them due to symptoms. In part it is the underground, unmonitored use of testosterone that creates so much bad publicity for this very helpful hormone.

The first step in the proper monitoring of replacement therapy is providing your doctor with a thorough medical history. Appendix A shows a simple and comprehensive medical history form (courtesy of Dr. John Crisler, allthingsmale.com). Patients who would like to be proactive can fill out this form and give a copy to their doctor. It is expected that every doctor have a similar form, although most do not ask questions pertinent to sexual function or on the use of androgens. Let your doctor know about all the medications you take so that medication-induced sexual dysfunction can be ruled out before starting testosterone.

I also strongly believe that if a patient goes to the doctor to obtain a Viagra, Cialis or Levitra prescription, the doctor should check the patient's testosterone and estradiol blood levels to ensure that abnormal levels of these two hormones are not the root cause of their ED. Hypogonadal men may not respond as well to ED drugs if their testosterone is not normalized first. Studies combining testosterone and oral sexual enhancement drugs have shown a synergistic effect on sexual benefits.

The following suggestions for monitoring testosterone replacement are recommended by several physician groups and practices:

1. You should be evaluated after the first month of therapy to measure your testosterone blood levels. If your doctor doesn't ask, let him/her know about your quality of life. Make sure

70

your doctor is aware of your energy level, mood, and sexual function, as well as any potential side effects (tender breasts, urinary flow decrease, frequent trips to the bathroom to urinate, moodiness, and acne).

2. When using testosterone, your doctor will want to measure total blood testosterone levels right before the next corresponding injection or gel use after the first month (it takes a while for the blood levels to stabilize). If testosterone is >900 ng/dl or <500 ng/dl, your doctor will adjust the amount or the frequency of your dose. I mentioned this earlier in the book but it bears repeating here: Some men need to have blood levels above 500 ng/dl to experience sexual function benefits from testosterone. It is important to be honest when your doctor asks you about your sexual performance. Do not let false pride, shame or machismo get in the way of a satisfying sexual and intimate life.

3. Your doctor should check your hematocrit before starting testosterone, after 3 months and then every year after that. If your hematocrit is above 52%, you should donate some blood in a blood bank or get a doctor's order for therapeutic phlebotomy if you cannot donate blood due to hepatitis or HIV (read the section "Checking for Increased Blood Thickness (Polycythemia)" or for more details. Usually, 4 units of blood can decrease hematocrit from 54 to 48 percent.

4. Be ready to have a digital rectal examination done and a prostatic specific antigen (PSA) blood test prior to starting testosterone, and after 3 months. Retesting every 6 months after that may not be unreasonable, especially in older men. A PSA above 4 ng/ml can be reason for concern and referral to an urologist. Testosterone replacement needs to be stopped if increases in PSA above normal are observed. Note: at the start of testosterone replacement in older men, when testosterone blood levels are rapidly rising, PSA may also increase. This is especially true when testosterone gels are employed, because they elevate DHT more relative to other options. Once testosterone levels have stabilized PSA drops back down to roughly baseline. It is important to allow "steady state" for testosterone fluctuations to stabilize before measuring PSA; a month or so should be sufficient. Also keep

72   *Nelson Vergel*
in mind that prostatic infections can also raise PSA, so it is
important to see an urologist to rule this out before deciding
to stop testosterone replacement due to high PSA.

5. If you start experiencing breast tenderness, pain or growth,
    ask your doctor to measure your estradiol blood level using
    the sensitive assay (not the regular test used for women).
    Normal range for estradiol in men is 14–54 pg/ml (50–200
    pmol/liter). Men who have high estradiol can be prescribed
    estrogen receptor inhibitors   (more details in "Avoiding
    enlarged breasts (gynecomastia")

I would like to stress that there is no agreement between several medical
guideline groups about the proper monitoring of TRT. And none of them
include estradiol measurement. You can see how each guideline group
recommends different schedules for monitoring testosterone, digital rectal
exam, prostatic specific antigen, and hematocrit. It is no wonder that
physicians in clinical practice are so confused about what is standard in
testosterone replacement therapy monitoring.

Table 4. Monitoring Testosterone Therapy

Monitoring testosterone therapy:
What the consensus guidelines say

q, every; BMD, bone mineral density; DRE, digital rectal exam; PSA, prostate-specific antigen

Organization	First follow-up	Digital Rectal Exam (DRE)	PSA test	Testosterone levels	Hematocrit	Bone Mineral Density	Lipids
American Association of Clinical Endocrinologist	q 3-4 mo in first year	q 6-12 mo	Annually		q 6 mo x 3, then annually	q 1-2 y	At 6-12 wk. then annually
American Society for Reproductive Medicines	At 2-3 mo	In first 2-3 mo	At 3 and 6 mo, then annually	At 3 and 6 mo, then annually	At 3 and 6 mo, then annually	At 2 y	
The Endocrine Society	At 3 mo. then annually	At 3 mo, then per routine guidelines	At 3 mo, then per routine guidelines	At 3 mo	At 3 mo, then annually	At 1-2 y	
European Association of Urology	At 3 mo	At 3 and 6 mo, then annually	At 3 and 6 mo, then annually		At 3 mo, then annually	q 1-2 y	

From: VOL 59, NO 12 | DECEMBER 2010 | THE JOURNAL OF FAMILY PRACTICE

Ensuring Prostate Health—No Link Found Between Androgen Levels and Risk for Prostate Cancer

The prostate is a gland that is part of the male reproductive system. Its function is to store and secrete a slightly alkaline (pH 7.29) a milky fluid which usually constitutes 25-30% of the volume of the semen along with spermatozoa. This alkaline fluid seems to neutralize the acidity in the vagina, prolonging the life span of the sperm. Also, the prostate contains some smooth muscles that help expel semen during ejaculation. It also helps control the flow of urine during ejaculation.

A healthy human prostate is classically said to be slightly larger than a walnut. In actuality, it is approximately the size of a kiwi fruit. It surrounds the urethra just below the urinary bladder and can be felt during a rectal exam. Refer to Figure 15 for more details on the prostate and surrounding organs.

Prostate cancer

This little gland attracts a great deal of attention in men's health. One of the major issues is related to cancer. Prostate cancer is one of the leading causes of death in men in the United States. As men age, small hidden prostatic lesions become increasingly common. These may or may not become cancerous. These lesions occur in 30 percent of American men over the age of 45, with the prevalence rising to more than 80 percent for men over the age of 80. Genetic factors and life style conditions such as diet are believed to contribute to this transformation.

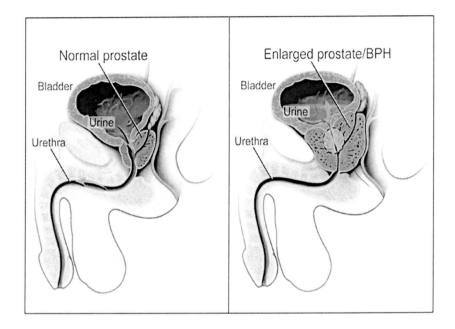

Figure 15. The prostate and surrounding organs

No association has been found between testosterone replacement therapy and prostate cancer. In 2004, a New England Journal of Medicine article review of over 60 studies on testosterone replacement therapy concluded that there is no causal or association with prostate cancer.

It is interesting to note that prostate cancer is most common in older men, the population known to have the highest incidence of low testosterone blood levels.

Doctors use different methods to detect prostate cancer, including prostate-specific antigen (PSA) assays, digital rectal examination (DRE), and transrectal ultrasound. A DRE before starting testosterone replacement therapy and every six months is recommended, especially for men with a family history of prostate cancer or those older than 40 years.   Nobody likes having a DRE but your continued good health is worth a few seconds of discomfort. An abnormal rectal exam, a confirmed increase in PSA greater than 2 ng/mL, or PSA of over 4 ng/mL will prompt a health care provider to refer you to a urologist for further evaluation (usually an ultrasound and prostate biopsies).

Admittedly the PSA and the DRE lack sensitivity and specificity. 25 percent of patients with prostate cancer have normal PSA levels (false negatives), while benign prostatic hyperplasia (BPH), a non-cancerous inflammation, may elevate them (false positives). Researchers have found hidden prostatic lesions with needle biopsies in some men with normal PSA level and normal transrectal ultrasound findings. Prostate biopsies are part of routine clinical use of testosterone therapy and are not justified unless a sharp rise in PSA is observed and infections have been ruled out.

Testosterone trials have inconsistently shown a rise in PSA, typically between 0.2 and 0.5 ng/mL. A greater increase in PSA arouses concern that prostate cancer has developed. Some physicians recommend a prostate biopsy in any patient with a yearly PSA increase of 1.0 ng/mL or more. If the PSA level increases by 0.75 ng/mL in one year, they repeat the PSA measurement in three to six months and recommend a biopsy if there is any further increase.

So, understandingly, there has some been confusion regarding testosterone replacement therapy's role in PSA elevation and prostate cancer. Prostate cancer is initially androgen-dependent so testosterone therapy should *not* be used by men with prostatic cancer. This does not mean that TRT causes cancer. A huge pooled analysis of data from 18 studies (consisting of 3,886 men with prostate cancer and 6,438 controls), published in the February 6, 2008 issue of the *Journal of the National Cancer Institute* found that blood levels of androgens and other sex hormones do not seem to be related to an increased risk for prostate cancer. In short, testosterone therapy does not appear to cause prostate cancer but it can make it worse if present at baseline.

Prostate infection

Another health concern is prostatitis or prostate infection. This is common in aging men and can be a leading cause of an elevated PSA. Your doctor will want to check you for an infection if your PSA unexpectedly increases by checking your urine for white blood cells. If they are high, he may refer you to an urologist who would induce a discharge from your penis to look at it under the microscope. Don't ask me how the urologist does it, ask the urologist!

Benign prostatic hyperplasia

A common health condition is benign prostatic hyperplasia or BPH. It is estimated to occur in 50 percent of men older than 50 years. Increased frequency of urination, frequent trips to the bathroom at night, incomplete voiding, and urgency to urinate indicate possible prostatic inflammation. BPH does not necessarily lead to increased rates of prostate cancer. There have been no prospective, controlled, long-term studies on the effects of testosterone administration on either the development or the progression of BPH. One open label, one-year study that measured prostate size using ultrasound found *no* increase during testosterone replacement therapy, suggesting that the treatment does not cause BPH. Whether testosterone treatment worsens asymptomatic BPH has not been established. However, some individuals are more prone to prostatic inflammation when using testosterone.

Another study (published in BJU International in December 2009) was conducted by Dr. Michael D. Trifiro at Moores UCSD Cancer Center in San Diego. Dr. Trifiro observed 158 men for 20 years to determine the correlation between serum sex hormones and lower urinary tract symptoms (reduced urinary flow, urgency, and other symptoms associated with BPH). The researchers found no significant associations of total testosterone, estradiol (E_2)), testosterone: E_2 ratio, DHT, or dehydroepiandrosterone with lower urinary track symptoms or with any measured hormones.

Testosterone replacement therapy is not contraindicated in those with BPH. Men with BPH who need to start testosterone replacement should be observed very closely. The first symptom that worsens with increased BPH is restricted urinary flow and urgency, especially during sleep hours. After ruling out prostatic infections and cancer, many urologists are successfully prescribing medications to improve urinary flow in men with BPH. Finasteride (brand name: Proscar), which was approved by the FDA in 1992, inhibits production of dihydrotestosterone (DHT), which may be involved with prostate enlargement. Its use can actually shrink the prostate in some men. However, many men using Proscar complain of erectile dysfunction (DHT receptors may be involved in healthy erections). For men who experience this side effect, other medications may be of help. Proscar has also been found to decrease the risk of prostate cancer in men by 25 percent over a seven year period. More studies are ongoing.

Another newer drug approved for BPH is dutasteride (brand name Avodart). Dutasteride, like finasteride, is in a class of medications called 5-alpha reductase inhibitors. This drug can also cause erectile dysfunction in men.

The FDA approved the drugs terazosin (brand name: Hytrin) in 1993, doxazosin (Cardura) in 1995, and tamsulosin (Flomax) in 1997 for the treatment of BPH. All three belong to the class of drugs known as alpha blockers. They work by relaxing the smooth muscle of the prostate and bladder neck to improve urine flow and to reduce bladder outlet obstruction. They do not seem to affect erectile dysfunction. In fact, they may improve erections in men with BPH.

Terazosin and doxazosin were developed first to treat high blood pressure. Tamsulosin is the first alpha-blocker developed specifically to treat BPH. The main side effects of these drugs are nasal congestion, lowered blood pressure, and rash or itching. Most men using them report fast improvements in their urine flow within one to three days. They end up not having to get up in the middle of the night to urinate, so they sleep better and feel less fatigued during the day.

The most common nonprescription agent used to alleviate symptoms of BPH is the over-the-counter herb saw palmetto (*Serenoa repens*). Extracted from the berry of the saw palmetto shrub, this substance is thought to inhibit 5-alpha reductase (5-R), thus blocking the conversion of testosterone into DHT, which is responsible for stimulating growth of the prostate gland.

Saw palmetto is generally well tolerated; side effects are infrequent, but include headache and gastrointestinal upset. No known drug interactions are associated with the use of this herb. Some studies found that saw palmetto led to an increase in urine flow rate in men with BPH compared with placebo, with effects comparable to finasteride.

One randomized, double-blind, placebo-controlled study followed men with BPH who took standardized saw palmetto extract 160 mg or placebo twice daily for one year. There was no significant difference found between the saw palmetto and placebo groups in standardized objective urinary symptoms. The incidence of side effects was similar in the two groups. These results cast considerable doubt on the effectiveness of saw palmetto for the treatment of BPH.

Patients who cannot tolerate BPH medications are now using emerging techniques like lasers to vaporize obstructing prostate tissue (www.greenlighthps.com). Talk to your urologist about this if you're interested. But be careful: This procedure can cause retrograde ejaculation since it may affect the bladder sphincter. Retrograde ejaculation occurs when semen, which would normally be ejaculated via the urethra, is redirected to the urinary bladder instead. Normally, the sphincter of the bladder contracts before ejaculation forcing the semen to exit via the urethra, the path of least pressure. When the bladder sphincter does not function properly, retrograde ejaculation may occur. This procedure may affect that sphincter. If you want to have children, I would suggest you do not use this technique.

PERSONAL COMMENT: After using testosterone for 17 years, I started to develop a weak urine flow. My doctor gave me prescriptions for several alpha blockers (Uroxatral, Flomax, etc). They worked great but I experienced a blistering rash with each one. My urologist found a prostate infection, which he treated with antibiotics. The infection seemed to linger for months. I then received an ultrasound of my prostate. This test showed that my prostate was not enlarged. Instead it showed that calcification, caused by a chronic prostatic infection, was blocking my urine flow through my prostate. I got the green light laser procedure done to open up my urethra. It worked great to enable normal urine flow. So, what may seem like BPH may not be! Prostatic infections often go untreated for months since in many cases we may not have symptoms.

Checking for Increased Blood Thickness (Polycythemia)

In addition to increasing muscle and sex drive, testosterone can increase your body's production of red blood cells. This hemopoietic (blood building) effect could be a good thing for those with mild anemia. An excessive production of red blood cells (erythrocytosis) is called polycythemia; it's not a good thing. With polycythemia the blood becomes very viscous or "sticky" making it harder for the heart to pump it. High blood pressure, strokes, and heart attacks can occur. This problem is not that common in men taking replacement doses of testosterone but more common in those taking higher bodybuilder doses.

It's important to have your doctor check your blood's hemoglobin and hematocrit. Hemoglobin is the substance that makes blood red and helps transport oxygen in the blood. Hematocrit reflects the proportion of red cells to total blood volume. The hemoglobin and hematocrit should be checked before starting testosterone replacement therapy, at three to six months and then annually. However, there is no agreement between medical guideline groups on this monitoring frequency, as shown in Table 4. A hematocrit of over 54 percent should be evaluated. Discontinuation of testosterone may be necessary but there is another option.

Polycythemia occurs quite frequently in people who are just on replacement testosterone. Older men appear more sensitive to the red blood cell enhancement effects of testosterone than young men do. Both testosterone dose and mode of delivery affect the degree of hematocrit elevation.

The incidence of testosterone-associated polycythemia may be lower in males using gels, patches and pellets, than it is in receiving intramuscular injections.

There seems to be a direct relation between testosterone dosage and the incidence of erythrocytosis (red blood cell increases). Erythrocytosis occurs in about 5– 15 percent by patches and in 10–20 percent with gel preparations depending on the use of 50 mg/day (delivering 5 mg /day) and 100 mg/day (delivering 10 mg/day) during the course of approximately 1 year.

Many patients on testosterone replacement who experience polycythemia do not want to stop the therapy due to fears of re-experiencing the depression, fatigue and low sex-drive they had before starting treatment. For those patients, therapeutic phlebotomy may be the answer. Therapeutic phlebotomy is very similar to what happens when donating blood, but this procedure is prescribed by your physician as a way to bring down your blood levels of hematocrit and viscosity. Of course, if you are a healthy man who has not been exposed to HIV and hepatitis, you can go to a blood bank to donate blood. This will decrease your hematocrit while you do something good for the world.

A phlebotomy of one pint of blood will generally lower hematocrit by about 3 percent. I have seen phlebotomy given every 3 months bring hematocrit from 56 percent to a healthy 46 percent. I know physicians who prescribe phlebotomy once every eight to ten weeks because of an unusual response to testosterone replacement therapy. This simple procedure is done in a hospital blood draw facility and can reduce hematocrit, hemoglobin, and blood iron easily and in less than one hour. Unfortunately, therapeutic phlebotomy can be a difficult option to get reimbursed or covered by insurance companies. Your doctor may need to write a letter of medical necessity for it.

The approximate amount of blood volume that needs to be withdrawn to restore normal hematocrit values can be calculated by the following formula, courtesy of Dr. Michael Scally, an expert on testosterone side effect management (read his interview later in this book). The use of the formula includes the assumption that whole blood is withdrawn. The duration over which the blood volume is withdrawn is affected by whether concurrent fluid replacement occurs.

Volume of Withdrawn Blood (cc) =

$$\text{Weight (kg)} \times ABV \times [Hgb_i - Hgb_f] / [(Hgb_i + Hgb_f)/2]$$

Where:

ABV = Average Blood Volume (default = 70)

Hgb_i (Hct_i) = Hemoglobin initial

Hgb_f (Hct_f) = Hemoglobin final (desired);

So, for a 70 kg (154 lbs) man (multiply lbs **x** 0.45359237 to get kilogram)

with an initial high hemoglobin of 20 mg/mL who needs to have it

brought down to a normal hemoglobin of 14 mg/mL, the calculation

would be:

CC of blood volume to be withdrawn = 75 **x** 70 **x** [20 — 14]/ [(20 +

14)/2]

= 75 **x** 70 **x** (6/17) = approximately 1850 cc;

   One unit of whole blood is around 350 to 450 cc; approximately 4
units of blood need to be withdrawn to decrease this man's hemoglobin
from 20 mg/mL to 14 mg/mL.
   The frequency of the phlebotomy depends on individual factors,
but most men can do one every two to three months to manage their
hemoglobin. Sometimes red blood cell production normalizes without any
specific reason. It is impossible to predict exactly who is more prone to
developing polycythemia, but men who use higher doses, men with higher
fat percentage, and older men may have a higher incidence.
   Some doctors recommend the use of a baby aspirin (81 mg) a day and
2,000 to 4,000 mg a day of omega-3 fatty acids (fish oil capsules) to help
lower blood viscosity and prevent heart attacks. These can be an important
part of most people's health regimen but they are not a replacement for
therapeutic phlebotomy if you have polycythemia and do not want to stop
testosterone therapy. It amazes me how many people assume that they are
completely free of stroke/heart attack risks by taking aspirin and omega-3
supplements when they have a high hematocrit.
   Although some people may have more headaches induced by high
blood pressure or get extremely red when they exercise, most do not feel
any different when they have polycythemia. This does not make it any
less dangerous. If you are using testosterone on your own you need to
let your doctor know. Your physician may already suspect some sort of
anabolic use if lab results reveal elevated hemoglobin and hematocrit.

PERSONAL COMMENT: I had polycythemia back in the mid-1990s
when I was using supraphysiologic doses of testosterone and nandrolone
to reverse my HIV-related weight loss. I required two phlebotomies in six
months. My hematocrit and hemoglobin eventually normalized without any

reason even when using the same doses of testosterone and nandrolone. So if you have polycythemia, it does not mean that you will have it forever in some cases.

Ensuring Liver Health

I mentioned this before but it is well worth repeating. Contrary to what some physicians may think, injectable and transdermal testosterone have *not* been known to cause increased liver enzymes. The same cannot be said for over-the-counter supplements that claim to increase testosterone or growth hormone. Not only do most of them not work, but they could increase your liver enzymes to dangerous levels. This problem has been reported in the past to the FDA. I warn people all the time to be careful about their use. It is always good to check your liver enzymes when blood work is done since it is a cheap test and highly useful in detecting toxicities caused by medications or supplements you may be using.

It is the use of oral testosterone and anabolic formulations (except for oral testosterone undecanoate, commonly used in Canada) that can increase liver enzymes. Many men with hepatitis B or C can be safely treated with replacement doses of testosterone without any liver injury if gels, patches or injections are used. I am very concerned that some of these patients may be denied this important therapy due to potential fears and misconceptions. Some studies have shown an increased incidence of hypogonadism, fatigue, and sexual dysfunction in patients with hepatitis.

Some men like to take supplements to protect the liver against the damaging effects of medications, but very limited data is available on their use. Supplements potentially can interfere with medication blood levels; very little is known about supplement-drug interactions. However, I would like to bring up some supplements with data on liver protection:

* Standardized silymarin (milk thistle herb)—160 mg/three times a day
* Evening primrose oil—1,300 mg/three times/day
* Alpha lipoic acid – 100 – 300 mg/three times/day
* Glycyrrhizinate Forte - Three or more capsules/day, but this may increase blood pressure.
* N-acetyl cysteine – 600 mg/three times/day
* Selenium – 200 mcg twice a day.

I trust the Jarrow and Super Nutrition brands for most of my supplements. Talk to your doctor before starting any supplements!

Monitoring Blood Pressure

High blood pressure or hypertension is another serious medical condition that can go undetected because it often has no symptoms. It's referred to as "the silent killer" for this reason. High blood pressure can cause heart attacks, strokes, headaches, ruin your kidneys, erectile dysfunction and shrink your brain.

Before you start testosterone replacement or an exercise program, it is very important to get your blood pressure under control. This is done through diet, stress management, lowering your salt intake and/or the use of medications. It is a good idea to invest in a home-based blood pressure machine. One usually can be purchased at most pharmacy chains and cost under $ 50. Some, like the OMRON HEM-780, can measure blood pressure easily and keep track of changes with time. Take measurements twice a day until you gain control of your blood pressure again.

Some men have higher conversions of testosterone into estradiol than others. High blood levels of estradiol can cause water retention, which can increase blood pressure. Polycythemia can also be one of the causes for increased blood pressure.

It is important to have your blood pressure measured during the first month of treatment to ensure that it does not increase with testosterone. The good news is that replacement doses are much less associated with this problem. More serious risks for hypertension are associated with the high testosterone doses associated with performance-enhancing use.

NOTE: Some natural ways to decrease blood pressure are decreasing your salt intake, exercising, keeping a normal body weight for your height, managing stress, and engaging in meditation and yoga. "Erection-friendlier" blood pressure medications like ACE (angiotensin converting enzyme) inhibitors, renin inhibitors, ARB's (angiotensin II receptor blockers), and combinations of them may be required for men who cannot maintain a blood pressure reading under 130/80 mm Hg. Diuretics, beta blockers, and calcium channel drugs used for hypertension may cause sexual dysfunction in men, but sometimes they cannot be avoided if your blood pressure cannot be controlled with ACE inhibitors or ARBs alone. Bu some studies show that blood pressure medications may be one of the main drug induced reasons for erectile dysfunction. But managing ED with drugs (read the corresponding section on ED options) is a healthier choice than allowing high blood pressure to go untreated due to fears of ED related side effects. Not only high blood pressure ensure that you have more cardiovascular risks, but it may also negatively affect your kidneys.

Avoiding Enlarged Breast (Gynecomastia)

Yes, I am talking about breast appearance in men, not women. Gynecomastia is a benign enlargement of the male breast resulting from a growth of the glandular tissue of the breast. It is defined clinically by the presence of a rubbery or firm mass extending concentrically from the nipples. Men who start experiencing this problem complain of pain and tenderness around the nipple area. Gynecomastia is caused by higher than normal blood levels of estradiol, a metabolite of estrogen. As discussed earlier in the book, testosterone can convert into estradiol, DHT, and other metabolites. Men with higher amounts of the enzyme aromatase usually have this problem even at lower doses of testosterone. Growth of this glandular tissue is influenced by a higher fat percentage, older age, excessive alcohol intake, and the use of certain medications. Gynecomastia usually occurs early in testosterone replacement in those who experience this side effect.

In several studies on testosterone replacement, only a very small percentage of people receiving testosterone experience growth of breast tissue. In one HIV-specific study conducted by Dr. Judith Rabkin in New York, she reported that out of 150 men enrolled in the study, two men experienced this adverse reaction. Gynecomastia is much more common among those who use high testosterone doses, such as bodybuilders (they call this "gyno").

How do you manage gynecomastia if it does occur? Lowering the testosterone dose had not proven helpful for the two patients in Dr. Rabkin's study. The use of antiestrogens, such as tamoxifen 10 mg twice daily, with lower doses of testosterone has been effective. Gynecomastia can become permanent if the condition lasts very long although it may reduce in size when the androgen use is discontinued. In the absence of resolution, surgical correction may be necessary in severe cases.

For men who experience enlarged breast size, doctors usually check estradiol levels to determine whether too much testosterone is being converted into estrogen. I do not believe that routine measurement of estrogen is needed for men who have no symptoms of high estrogen (mainly breast tissue enlargement and water retention). For those who have higher than normal estrogen, doctors usually prescribe an antiestrogen medication. One such regimen is anastrozole at 1 mg/day during the first week until nipple soreness and breast enlargement disappear. The dose is then lowered to 0.25 mg a day, or 1 mg twice a week.

A warning: Bringing estrogen down to very low levels could cause health problems in men in the long run. Hair/skin quality and health, brain function, bone density, and other important factors may be greatly influenced by estrogen. However a 12-week study in men using anastrozole at 1 mg a day and 1 mg twice a week found no changes in bone metabolism markers.

The normal production ratio of testosterone to estrogen is approximately 100:1. The normal ratio of testosterone to estrogen in the circulation is approximately 300:1. Estrogen (measured as estradiol) should be kept at 30 picograms per milliliter (pg/mL) or lower. As men grow older or as they gain a lot of fat mass, their estrogen blood levels increase, even to levels higher than that of postmenopausal women. But estrogen is important for men's health, so decreasing it to levels less than 20 pg/dl may not be a smart idea.

Medications and Products That Can Cause Gynecomastia

A number of medications have been reported in the medical literature to cause gynecomastia due to decreases in testosterone, increases in estradiol, or both. These include:

- Antiandrogens. These include cyproterone, flutamide, and finasteride. Used to treat prostate cancer and some other conditions.
- HIV medications. Sustiva, Atripla, and Videx have been associated with gynecomastia.
- Anti-anxiety medications such as diazepam (Valium).
- Tricyclic antidepressants. These include amitriptyline.
- Glucocorticoid steroids.
- Antibiotics.
- Ulcer medication such as cimetidine (Tagamet).
- Cancer treatment (chemotherapy).
- Heart medications such as digitalis and calcium channel blockers.
- Anabolic steroids

Substances that have been reported to cause gynecomastia include:
- AlcoholAmphetamines
- Marijuana
- Heroin
- Soy and flaxseed- There are conflicting studies but it is something to keep in mind
- Exposure to pesticides and byproducts of plastic processing has also been linked to increased estrogen and decreased sperm count in men.

Does Testosterone Suppress the Immune System?

This question is raised out of the confusion over the use of the term "steroid." When somebody is having pain or inflammation and their physician prescribes them a "steroid" or something "steroidal", they are prescribing a corticosteroid (like prednisone) to decrease inflammation. These can have an immunosuppressive effect (sometimes it is intended to decrease inflammation). The "steroid" that you hear about from the media when they are talking about use and abuse by athletes refers to an anabolic steroid (like testosterone). The similarities largely end with their street names.

Some *in vitro* and animal data do suggest that high dose testosterone could be immune suppressive. No such immunosuppressive effect is seen when testosterone was added at replacement concentrations. Several studies using testosterone alone or on combination with oxandrolone or nandrolone in HIV-positive immune compromised patients have found no immune suppressive effect. Testosterone has been used in HIV since 1992 without any reports of immune related problems.

PERSONAL COMMENT: I have lived with immune dysfunction for 27 years and testosterone has not worsened it. In fact, it may have helped me retain the mood, appetite, and muscle mass needed for good immune function.

Protecting your Heart and Keeping Cholesterol (Lipids) in Check

There is widespread misinformation that testosterone supplementation increases the risk of heart disease. There is no evidence to support this in men younger than 65 years of age. In fact testosterone administration to middle-aged men is actually associated with decreased visceral fat, triglycerides, lower blood sugar concentrations and increased insulin sensitivity. Several studies have shown that low total and free testosterone concentrations are linked to increased intra-abdominal fat mass, risk of coronary artery disease, and type 2 diabetes mellitus. Testosterone has also been shown to increase coronary blood flow. Similarly, testosterone replacement retards the build-up of plaque in experimental models of atherosclerosis.

In 1994, Phillips and colleagues studied 55 men with angina. They found a strong correlation between very low levels of testosterone and increased severity of coronary artery disease as measured by arteriograms, suggesting that testosterone may actually have a protective effect. This is consistent with the observation that the risk for atherosclerosis increases with age in men, while testosterone levels decrease. Two other smaller studies found that the administration of testosterone decreased risk factors for coronary artery disease.

The European prospective investigation into cancer in Norfolk (EPIC-Norfolk) Prospective Population Study examined the prospective relationship between the body's own (endogenous) testosterone concentrations and mortality due to all causes, cardiovascular disease, and cancer in a nested case-control study based on 11,606 men aged 40 to 79 years surveyed in 1993 to 1997 and followed up to 2003. Among those without prevalent cancer or cardiovascular disease, 825 men who subsequently died were compared with a control group of 1489 men still alive, matched for age and date of baseline visit. Lower endogenous testosterone (the body's own) concentrations at baseline were linked to mortality due to all causes (825 deaths), cardiovascular disease (369 deaths), and cancer (304 deaths). So this study found that in men, endogenous testosterone concentrations are inversely related to mortality due to cardiovascular disease and all causes, and that low testosterone may be a predictive marker for those at high risk of cardiovascular disease.

But there is some emerging contradicting data from a much smaller study that showed that older men who have higher endogenous testosterone (without taking testosterone) may have a higher incidence of heart disease. A large U.S. multicenter study showed that older men with higher testosterone levels are more likely to have a heart attack or other cardiovascular disease in the future. The results were presented at The Endocrine Society's 92nd Annual Meeting in San Diego in June 2010. Study participants were age 65 or older and included 697 community-dwelling men who were participating in the National Institutes of Health-funded study, called the Osteoporotic Fractures in Men (MrOS). None of these men were receiving testosterone therapy, according to the study abstract.

All subjects had blood tests to determine their testosterone levels. The investigators then divided the men into quartiles, or four groups, of testosterone range to observe trends in rates of coronary heart disease events. This type of heart disease results from plaque-clogged or narrowed coronary arteries, also called atherosclerosis. A coronary heart disease event included a heart attack; unstable angina, which is chest pain usually due to atherosclerosis and which doctors consider a prelude to a heart attack; or an angioplasty or bypass surgery to clear blocked arteries.

During an average follow-up of nearly 4 years, 100 men, or about 14 percent, had a coronary disease event, in particular, heart attacks. After the researchers adjusted for other potential contributing risk factors for heart disease, such as elevated cholesterol, they found that higher total testosterone level relates to an increased risk of coronary disease. Men whose total testosterone was in the highest quartile (greater than or equal to 495 nanograms per deciliter, or ng/dL) had more than twofold the risk of coronary disease compared with men in the lowest quartile (below 308 ng/dL). So, this is contradictory data that may be concerning, but does it say anything about the cardiovascular risks of supplementing testosterone to men with testosterone deficiency?

A report published in the New England Journal of Medicine in June 2010 about a study researching the use of testosterone gel in older men showed that such study was stopped early due to a higher incidence of side effects in men treated with the gel. Participants in this trial called the Testosterone in Older Men with Mobility Limitations, or TOM, were non-institutionalized men aged 65 and older who had difficulty walking two blocks or climbing 10 steps and whose serum testosterone was 100 to 350 ng/dl (very low levels). So, these were frail older men. The goal was to recruit 252 men, but only 209 subjects had been enrolled by the time the trial, which started in 2005, was stopped on December 2010. Testosterone use had the desired effect of improving the men's muscle strength and mobility. But they also experienced a high rate of adverse effects — not just cardiovascular problems but respiratory and skin problems. Unfortunately, they did not report hematocrit, estradiol and bio available testosterone. I dream of the day when a study will be done the right way to include all of those variables. Only then we can draw the right conclusions about who is more prone to side effects. Managing high hematocrit with blood donation/phlebotomy and high estradiol with anastrazole can probably eliminate some of the reported side effects in older men, but there really is only one way to find out: To have proper studies using those management strategies. To date, no study listed in clinicaltrials.gov is actually following men who are taking testosterone and who have access to phlebotomy or estrogen blockers to manage the two main side effects that may affect cardiovascular health in older men: high hematocrit and estradiol.

Previous studies have shown that in general, older men have more side effects when using testosterone (polycythemia, gynecomastia, high blood pressure, prostatic hyperplasia) and more co morbid conditions. High hematocrit and estradiol increase clotting and viscosity, so it is not surprising to me that older men who use testosterone would have more cardiovascular risks if monitored poorly by their physicians. It amazes me how many older men using TRT are walking around with hematocrit over 54 and estradiol levels above 100 pg/dl without being offered phlebotomy or estrogen blockers. This is one of the main reasons I felt compelled to write this book.

Older men also require more testosterone to reach normal levels since they have more sex hormone binding globulin that attaches to testosterone and renders it useless. So, physicians should carefully monitor these patients if they decide to provide testosterone replacement. The age cut off when the risk-to-benefit ratio of testosterone changes is not known yet. There are several studies listed in the Appendix that are currently being performed to provide more answers.

So, the jury is still out. But if no complicating factors like high cholesterol, blood pressure or strong family history of heart disease are present, many doctors opt for prescribing testosterone to older men who need it to have a better quality of life. And most doctors keep an eye on hematocrit but few on estradiol. Hopefully, this will change as more doctors wake up to the risks associated with poor monitoring and management of TRT.

It is the excessively high doses of testosterone used by athletes and recreational body builders that are linked to significant decreases in the plasma concentration of HDL (high-density lipoprotein - the good cholesterol) and increases in LDL (low-density lipoprotein – the bad cholesterol). Replacement doses of testosterone have been shown to have only a modest or no effect on plasma HDL in placebo-controlled trials. Testosterone supplementation has been show to decrease triglycerides, a dissolved fat that can lead to cholesterol increases and metabolic syndrome. In spite of these studies, some physicians continue to think that testosterone replacement can dramatically increase cholesterol levels.

Given the state of the modern diet, all of us should have our doctor check our fasting cholesterol and triglycerides (another lipid linked with heart disease risk). If you think that you have low testosterone you may already have a problem with your lipids. The recommendations of exercise and diet (low in sugars and animal fats) apply for everybody but are especially important for men who have high LDL and high triglycerides at the time of starting testosterone replacement. Testosterone therapy can be an important part of your health regimen but don't start it thinking that it will cure high cholesterol. Sometimes high lipids are related to poor diet, sedentary lifestyle, medication side effects, and/or bad genes. Your treatment for high cholesterol and triglycerides can also include statin and fibrates drugs prescribed to you by your doctor. I would try to modify your diet and to exercise before you jump on taking these medications since they may have muscle related side effects and really do not correct the root cause of the problem, which is a metabolic abnormality that could be addressed with good adherence to life style modifications. The key word is "adherence", which seems elusive is many people who rather take a pill than watch their diet and exercise. For more on diet and exercise, refer to the chapter "Miscellaneous Health Tips to Support Healthy Testosterone."

NOTE: I think you're getting why I'm telling you that you need doctor's supervision when on testosterone. So far you've read about the potential impact on hemoglobin and hematocrit, blood pressure, and estradiol, all of which can negatively affect your cardiovascular health. Imagine the even greater risk of those using testosterone at higher than replacement doses that usually buy it from underground sources and do not have a doctor who monitors them. No wonder testosterone and anabolic steroids get such bad reputation. I tell bodybuilders that do not have a doctor to follow them to at least decrease their risks by getting blood work done in independent labs that do not require a prescription. There are many around the United States and you can find them by googling "blood tests no prescription + your zip code". Of course, this is not the best solution and in no way a replacement for the supervision of a doctor. Irresponsible bodybuilders do more self-inflicted damage when their mistakes fuel the hysteria surrounding hormones in the United States. This hysteria has made it difficult for many men who need TRT to get it.

Over-the-counter "testosterone boosters" may problems with lipids, so do not think that because you are buying something at a health food store, that makes that product safe. Let your doctor know if you are taking any of those. Most do not work and those that did where banned by the FDA and taken off the market. Some have been found to have generic Arimidex from China. For more information on them, refer to the chapter 5.

Azoospermia (low sperm count)

Sperm are the male reproductive cells found in semen. One possible side effect of testosterone replacement is azoospermia or low sperm count. This can mean infertility and is of course an issue if you want to have children.

Adding supraphysiological (above normal) testosterone to the body shuts down sperm production so much that the administration of testosterone injections as a means of male contraception is under study. In study participants azoospermia usually results within approximately 10 weeks of beginning therapy. Rebound of the sperm count to baseline levels occurs within 6 to 18 months of cessation, and subsequent fertility has been demonstrated.

However, studies have shown that a large proportion of men do not suffer significant decreases in sperm count with replacement doses of testosterone, especially if gels are used. But it is always a good idea for men who want to have children and are on testosterone replacement to consult their urologist. Some of these men may need to discontinue testosterone and wait for their sperm production to normalize if their sperm count is found to be low for impregnating a woman. For men who cannot normalize their sperm count after a few weeks or months of testosterone cessation, a combination of HCG and other gonadotropin hormones may be required.

Some fertility doctors prescribe subcutaneous injections of gonadotropin releasing hormone (GnRH) (brand names: Factrel, Lutepulse) alone to increase sperm production. They may also prescribe a combination of HCG at a dose of 1000-2500 IU twice a week plus 75-150 IU of human menopausal gonadotropin (HMG) (brand name: Pergonal or Repodex) three times a week. HMG is a hormone extracted from menopausal women that mimics FSH. Other FSH-like hormones that have been used in place of HMG are human urinary follicle stimulating hormone (Brand name: Fertinex) or recombinant FSH (Brand name: Follistin). As mentioned before, FSH stimulates sperm production in the presence of normal levels of LH and testosterone. These protocols have been able to induce normal sperm production in 5-9 months, so it is important to adhere to it for this long period of time before potential fertility can occur. As you can see, fertility enhancement in men with low sperm counts is a complex issue that needs to be monitored by a qualified fertility physician.

Moodiness

Most people are familiar with the term "roid rage." It is a phenomenon that is occasionally seen among athletes who may be using up to 100 times the medically recommended doses of anabolics and who typically combine several different steroids at once. It usually refers to responses of much greater than expected aggression. For some the term conjures up images of a vein-popping Hulk-like character going on a rampage. Some people unfairly expect this result with any use of testosterone, regardless of the dose used.

In a 1994 study by Drs. Harrison Pope and David Katz, published in the *Archives of General Psychiatry* 88 athletes who were steroid users were compared with 68 non-users. Among the men using high doses (defined as more than 1,000 mg of anabolic steroids/week), manic as well as hypomanic episodes were reported, in addition to episodes of major depression. In contrast the non-users or athletes using "low" doses (less than 300 mg/week) experienced no manic or depressive episodes. They concluded that psychiatric effects are subtle at physiologic doses but become more prominent at supraphysiologic (above normal) doses.

The testosterone researcher Dr. James Dabbs, studied 692 prison inmates to see whether their natural testosterone levels matched their aggression levels. He wrote, "Aggression is only part of the overall picture relating testosterone to behavior. Connections between testosterone and aggression or other antisocial behavior are very much moderated by social forces." He said that he prefers the term, "rambunctiousness," which suggests in a more neutral manner an increase in overall energy and assertiveness.

In another study by Dr. Judith Rabkin, HIV-positive men with low testosterone were given testosterone supplementation. She observed no major mood effects, but did note increases in self-reported irritability. In fact, this was the side effect most commonly reported in her study: 19 percent (28/150) of the patients noticed that they were uncharacteristically assertive, bossy, "hyper," and/or more prone to anger during the first 12 weeks of treatment. However this was a transient effect for most; only 6 of the 28 reported increased irritability on two consecutive visits. This was seldom a cause for concern to the patient.

Dr. C. Wang and colleagues from the University of California-Harbor performed a study to assess the effects of testosterone replacement on changes in mood in 51 hypogonadal men for 60 days. They concluded that testosterone replacement therapy in these men improved their positive mood parameters, such as energy, well/good feelings, and friendliness and decreased negative mood parameters including anger, nervousness, and irritability.

So, it seems that depending on the study that you read, testosterone can improve mood or increase rambunctiousness.

PERSONAL COMMENT: I feel my best when my total testosterone is between 500-1000 ng/dL (mid to upper normal range). My coping mechanisms, outlook, energy level, mental focus, connection to others and productivity are great. Only when I have let testosterone drop is when all of those mood parameters drastically change for the worse (I become more negative in my thinking, more irritable, more fatigued, and don't want to deal with small tasks like calling people back). But we are all different in our response to medicines. I have never had a problem with high estradiol, which has also been linked to moodiness.

Acne and Baldness

We usually associate acne with our teen years when our testosterone levels were off the chart and balding as part of getting older. As I mentioned earlier, some testosterone is converted into DHT (dihydrotestosterone). Acne is caused by DHT's stimulating effect on the skin's sebaceous glands; too much oil and sebum are produced and can get infected with bacteria. Hair thinning and balding is caused by DHT's negative effect on the hair follicles.

Patients with mild acne and/or a history of adolescent acne may experience eruptions with testosterone therapy, especially on the back and shoulders.

Dr. Judith Rabkin in New York City studied 150 HIV-positive men who were treated in an open study for 12 weeks with testosterone. Acne was reported by 8 percent (12/150), in one instance leading to study discontinuation.

There are various ways of managing acne.

- Taking a shower right after a workout and using a body scrubbing brush can help remove the excess oil induced by higher DHT.

- Antibacterial soaps (such as Lever 2000) or acne prevention washes and creams with benzoyl peroxide or salicylic acid can also help.

- Getting sun exposure for at least 20 minutes a day seems to benefit some people.

- There are studies that show that taking 50 mg of zinc (plus 3 mg of copper to balance it) can decrease the incidence of acne.

- If acne is related to an infection, some doctors might prescribe antibiotics (erythromycin topical solution USP, 2 percent, and/or erythromycin 250 mg twice a day is often helpful).

- The use of prescription acne medications like isotretinoin (Accutane) should be done under strict medical supervision since it has been linked to liver problems and mood fluctuations. It can also lower testosterone blood levels permanently.

- **NOTE:** Other skin problems in HIV-positive patients, particularly folliculitis, may be confused with acne, but are not related to testosterone levels.

Men who are already losing hair (male pattern baldness or related to a health condition) are most likely to experience hair loss with testosterone therapy. Hair loss was reported by 6 percent of the men during the first 12 weeks of testosterone treatment in one small study. Hair loss seems to stabilize after the 30's, though, so it is unlikely that testosterone replacement can increase this problem after a certain age. And some people seem to be resistant to any DHT, so genetics have a strong influence of who keep their hair as they age.

There are a few options for managing hair loss. Propecia (finasteride, the same drug we previously discussed in the prostate section) is a prescription medication approved for hair loss, more cheaply available as the generic finasteride. Some men have reported erectile problems with this medication since it tends to decrease DHT action. DHT is needed for proper erectile function.

Rogaine® lotion is an over-the-counter product that may be of benefit; it is available at most stores. Nizoral®, an anti-dandruff shampoo available as a prescription and over-the-counter at a lower concentration, may help out too. It wasn't originally intended for this purpose but it seems to help block DHT's effect on hair follicles.

PERSONAL COMMENT: I really like a product called OC Eight when my face gets too oily (available on amazon.com). I take zinc every day and have never had an acne issue even when using anabolics with testosterone in the past. My hair is another story. I lost a lot of it while using an HIV medication called Crixivan that was later found to cause this and many other problems. Testosterone has not caused any more loss after that. I use Nizoral shampoo three times a day since there may be some evidence that it helps protect against DHT's effect on hair follicles. I formulated a over-the-counter hair gel called Regenase with a combination of minoxinyl and ketoconazole that I used to get compounded.

Testicular Shrinkage (Atrophy) and Decreased Ejaculate

Testicular atrophy and decreased ejaculate (amount of semen produced by a man when he climaxes) are common with aging. They also occur in approximately 20 percent of men on long-term testosterone therapy (six months or more). Also, some men may have retrograde ejaculation as they age as their prostate sphincter malfunctions and sends the sperm to the bladder instead of forward towards the gland. There are no effective treatments for this problem.

One helpful treatment for these side effects is the administration of HCG. I've discussed this thoroughly under the section on HCG so I will keep it brief here. HCG stimulates the testicles to retain their size and function while making testosterone. HCG administration is done either as a subcutaneous (under the skin) or intramuscular (into the muscle) injection, both equally effective. A single weekly injection seems sufficient to offset testicular atrophy, although for other conditions HCG is administered several times a week. Many physicians prescribe testosterone injections at a dose of 100 to 200 mg a week with 500 to 1000 IU of HCG weekly.

Some urologists have asked patients to estimate their previous testicular size using an orchidometer (Genentech Inc.), and then measured testicular change with HCG treatment. A return to original size has occurred.

PERSONAL COMMENT: HCG works for sure to increase testicular size. I started using it twice a week at 250 IU per injection but later found out that one injection a week was good enough to keep my testicles feel full again. I really TRT plus HCG, although there are no data showing what doses and injection frequency are best. I get my HCG by prescription cheaply from compounding pharmacies listed on TestosteroneWisdom. com since the pharmaceutical products are a rip off when it comes to price. Most insurance companies refuse to pay for HCG to maintain testicular size while on testosterone replacement. I will provide more information on HCG in chapter 3 and the following section.

Hypothalamic-Pituitary-Gonadal Axis (HPGA) Dysfunction

If you do a quick review of Figure 1 back in chapter 2 and of the sections on HCG and Clomid in chapter 3 you will remember that low testosterone is caused by a problem somewhere in the HPG axis (also called HPT axis). I am adding Figure 1 here again for the purpose of explaining one of the most important and neglected side effects of using testosterone or anabolic steroids.

What you also need to know is that testosterone replacement therapy itself can lead to further HPGA dysfunction. Supplemental testosterone can inhibit the release of the body's own testosterone production through negative feedback inhibition on LH levels. This feedback inhibition also results in suppression of FSH levels, leading to suppression of sperm production (spermatogenesis).

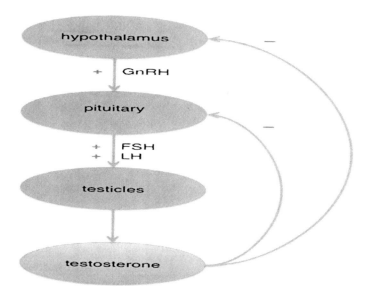

Figure 1. HPG axis

Some men need to stop using testosterone or other androgens because side effects are a problem (e.g. low sperm count interferes with their goal to have children). Most physicians advise the patient to just stop testosterone without thinking about the possible consequences of the hypogonadal state after treatment cessation. Will the patient be worse off than when he started?

Not all studies show a shutdown of the HPGA in patients after testosterone cessation. In a study previously mentioned in the Moodiness section, Dr. Rabkin compiled data for 42 patients who were treated with testosterone for 12 weeks and then randomized (double blind) to receive placebo injections for six weeks. At week 13 (one week after their first placebo injection and three weeks since the last active injection), mean testosterone level was 286 ng/dL. At week 15 (after 2 placebo injections), mean testosterone level was 301, and after week 17 (after 3 placebo injections), mean serum level was 324 ng/dL. None of these values was statistically different from the mean baseline testosterone level of 308 ng/dL. These data suggest that for men who were already hypogonadal there was no further decline in the body's production of testosterone once testosterone therapy was discontinued after 12 weeks of use. It is not known if longer term testosterone use would have the same results.

When high-dose testosterone use (as in bodybuilding) is discontinued the HPGA dysfunction that occurs when it is stopped may be a lot more pronounced. Stopping treatment may cause the patient to suffer all the symptoms of hypogonadism for weeks or months. Many lose a lot of the muscle mass they gained through their cycle of anabolics plus testosterone. In some cases a specific medical protocol is required for HPGA normalization. If you go to bodybuilding sites, you will see Clomid and HCG mentioned a lot for this purpose.

There is no controlled data from studies using any protocols to accelerate the normalization of normal testosterone production in men who have used either supplemented physiologic (normal) or supraphysiologic (above normal) doses of testosterone for long periods.

For men who had normal testosterone before starting testosterone or anabolic steroids (athletes, bodybuilders or certain people with wasting syndrome) and who want or need to stop those compounds, some physicians have attempted to jump-start testicular testosterone production using a combination of products that have different effects on the HPGA and estrogen receptors. One such physician is Dr. Michael Scally from Houston (read the interview in Chapter 7) who presented a poster at the Lipodystrophy and Adverse Reactions in HIV conference in San Diego in 2002 that reported the use of a protocol to normalize testosterone production in HIV-positive patients after prolonged anabolic steroid and testosterone use for their wasting syndrome.

The protocol consisted of the use of HCG, clomiphene citrate, and tamoxifen (read about each of these products in their respective sections). Treatment takes place over two discrete intervals. The first treatment interval is to initiate the restoration of gonadal function. The second interval is to restore the hormonal pathways among the hypothalamus, the pituitary and the gonads. The medications are initiated simultaneously after cessation of androgens when it is expected that the body would try to start to slowly make its own testosterone. If the testosterone ester (cypionate, enanthate, undecanoate, Sustanon) that the patient used is known (the most common one in the United States is depo testosterone or testosterone cypionate), its half-life in the body can be estimated so that the date to begin the medical protocol can be predicted with some accuracy to assess a time when no pharmaceutical testosterone remains in the body.

The protocol for HPTA normalization contains:

First 15 days:

   HCG 2,500 IU (subcutaneous) once every other day;

Clomiphene citrate 50 mg orally twice a day; and

Tamoxifen 20 mg orally once a day.

A satisfactory testosterone level on day 15, typically 350 ng/mL or greater, is followed by the oral medications (no HCG) for an **additional 15 days**.

This protocol has not been tested in many patients but has shown good results in restoring HPGA in a month. I know that this sounds like a long time but without treatment the body's restoration process would take about the same length of time that somebody was using androgens. In some, HPGA function and testosterone production never returns to normal. Hopefully we will see data on approaches like this one used in patients who need to stop testosterone or anabolics after long term use. However, no such studies are listed in clinicaltrials.gov.

Most doctors will refuse to prescribe the protocol above since they are not familiar with it. But remember that this protocol will likely not help most men who had low testosterone before starting TRT anyway. It is more likely to be helpful to those who used testosterone and anabolics for muscle building purposes and who were not hypogonadal before starting their muscle building cycles.

-5-

When Testosterone is Not Enough

When Testosterone Replacement Doesn't Lead to Better Erections and More Energy

Most men find that their sexual desire increases after they start testosterone replacement. Sexual dreams and nighttime/morning erections may be more easily achievable, but in some cases testosterone alone does not make erections strong or lasting enough for successful intercourse. So, some men need some extra help to make sure that their improved sex drive matches an improved and hard erection.

Before we start covering other options for improving erections, let's talk about steps you should take before you start combination therapy of testosterone plus other options. If erectile dysfunction or sex drive is not improved while on testosterone, ask your doctor about adjusting your dose of testosterone. Ensure that your total testosterone level is between 500 and 1000 ng/dL. Also, have your doctor check your blood levels of estradiol. High estradiol blood levels caused by conversion of testosterone into this female hormone by the aromatase enzyme may cause sexual dysfunction (this can be treated with low dose anastrazole). Low levels of thyroid hormone, infections, lack of sleep, alcohol, smoking, medications and depression also can cause erectile dysfunction in the presence of normal testosterone levels. Blood pressure medications are known to be one of the main causes of erectile dysfunction, so discuss the different type of medications to keep your blood pressure in normal ranges (high blood pressure is also a risk factor for erectile dysfunction). Last but not least, lack of attraction for our sexual partner can get in the way of achieving a strong erection.

HCG- As mentioned before, human chorionic gonadotropin (HCG) mimics LH and stimulates the Leydig cells of the testicles to produce testosterone. HCG has been successfully used alone or in combination with testosterone replacement to normalize testicular size after long term anabolic steroid or testosterone use. It has also anecdotally helped men whose sexual drive does not improve on testosterone replacement alone. No published studies have been done on this benefit, however. Doses of 250-500 IU twice a week while on testosterone replacement are being prescribed by several physicians who report that their patients perceive improvements in sexual desire and erectile function on this regimen. We do not know if this effect lasts after long term HCG use or if it is better to cycle it on and off.

PD-5 Inhibitors- For many older men the use of prescription phosphodiesterase type 5 inhibitor (PD-5) medications like *Viagra, Cialis, and Levitra*—may be needed in combination with testosterone replacement. However, some men do not respond well to these oral agents or have side effects such as headaches, nasal congestion, flushing, gut problems, and, in the case of Cialis, back pain. Cialis may last longer than the others (36 hours compared to 4 hours for Viagra or Levitra), but so may its side effects. Some men take Claritin and ibuprofen with these drugs to pre-treat nasal congestion and headaches, respectively.

Sildenafil (Viagra) was the first PDE5 inhibitor to enter on the market in 1998. The usual dose of sildenafil is 50 mg (25 to 100 mg) taken one hour before sex. The effects of sildenafil last for approximately four hours, and patients should be instructed to use no more than one dose within 24 hours. Fatty meals reduce the absorption of sildenafil; therefore, the drug should be taken on an empty stomach. This may be an inconvenient factor that needs careful planning of which some patients are not aware.

Vardenafil (Levitra), the first second-generation PDE5 inhibitor to be developed, is given at a usual dose of 10 mg (2.5 to 20 mg) one hour before sex. Older men and those with moderate liver dysfunction should receive a lower initial dose of 5 mg. Vardenafil begins working within 30 to 45 minutes after administration and lasts for about four hours. As with sildenafil, patients taking vardenafil should not use more than one dose within a 24-hour period. Patients should not take vardenafil within three hours of fatty meals, due to a reduction in absorption.

The newest PDE5 inhibitor is tadalafil (Cialis), which has a longer duration of action--approximately 36 hours--than sildenafil or vardenafil. In addition, the usual dose of 10 mg (5 to 20 mg) should be taken about 30 minutes before sexual activity. This shorter onset time can possibly allow patients more opportunity for spontaneity. Food intake does not appear to affect the absorption of tadalafil; this makes it very practical for men who do not plan ahead when they have sex. Cialis is approved for low dose daily use, but most insurance companies will not pay for it. If you want to try a 5 or 10 mg dose daily, you can get a free 30 day supply after getting a doctor's prescription and taking the following voucher to your pharmacy after downloading it and printing it (you have to answer some questions online first). You are better off asking your doctor for a prescription for 10 mg per day and cut the pills in half for the first week to see if 5 mg per day works well enough for you. If not, you can go up in dose. Here is the web site address to download the voucher:

voucher.cialis.com/index.cfm

Though considered generally safe for most patients, including those taking multiple antihypertensives, PDE5 inhibitors are not a viable treatment option for every man with ED. They need to be used with careful monitoring in patients with a cardiovascular history that includes heart attacks or stroke (within the past two weeks) and hypotension (blood pressure <90/50 mmHg),

Because PDE5 is inhibited in penile tissue as well as extra genital tissue, patients treated with PDE5 inhibitors may experience headache, facial flushing, nasal congestion, dyspepsia, and dizziness. Sildenafil also inhibits PDE type 6 in the retina. Therefore, patients treated with sildenafil may experience sensitivity to light, blurred vision, and loss of blue-green color discrimination, all of which are generally considered reversible. Tadalafil also inhibits PDE type 11 in skeletal tissue, possibly leading to back and muscle pain.

ED drugs are available by prescription but I have heard that some men are ordering them without a prescription from overseas websites to save money (overseas sources can be ten times cheaper than products in the United States). This book does not endorse the use of these drugs without a prescription, but it is my duty to mention facts about what is happening out in the real world. For a review of online sites that sell erectile dysfunction drugs, visit:

www.edguider.com/ed_pharmacies/list/onecat/ed_pharmacies/0. html

The following table shows how long each commercially available PD-5 drug starts working and how long they stay in your body. This numbers vary depending on the amount of food or alcohol you ingest before taking them, your body weight, and your liver metabolism.

Table 5. Erectile Dysfunction Oral Drugs

Erectile Dysfunction Oral Drugs
How long do they start working and how long do they stay in your body?

Drug	Onset of Action	Duration of Activity	Available Doses
Viagra	60 minutes	4-5 hours	25, 50 and 100 mg
Levitra	30 minutes	4-5 hours	2.5, 5, 10 and 20 mg
Cialis*	15 minutes	36 hours	5, 10 and 20 mg

* No food effect (you can take it with or without food). Food lengthens time to onset of action of the other two options.

If you are older than age 65, or have serious liver or kidney problems, your doctor may start you at the lowest dose (25 mg) of Viagra or any of the other two drugs.

Tell your doctor about all the medicines you take. ED drugs and other medicines may affect each other. Especially tell your doctor if you take any of these:

- Medicines called alpha-blockers. These include Hytrin® (terazosin HCl), Flomax® (tamsulosin HCl), Cardura® (doxazosin mesylate), Minipress® (prazosin HCl), Uroxatral® (alfuzosin HCl), or Rapaflo® (silodosin). Alpha-blockers are sometimes prescribed for prostate problems or high blood pressure. In some patients the use of PDE5 inhibitor drugs with alpha-blockers can lower blood pressure significantly, leading to fainting. You should contact the prescribing physician if alpha-blockers or other drugs that lower blood pressure are prescribed by another healthcare provider

- HIV protease inhibitors including Ritonavir (Norvir®) or indinavir sulfate (Crixivan®), saquinavir (Fortavase® or Invirase®) or atazanavir (Reyataz®)

- Antifungals like ketoconazole or itraconazole (such as Nizoral® or Sporanox®)

- Antibiotics like erythromycin or clarithromycin

- Tell your doctor if you take medicines that treat abnormal heartbeat. These include quinidine, procainamide, amiodarone, and sotalol. Patients taking these drugs should not use ED drugs.

If you are taking HIV protease inhibitors your doctor may recommend the lowest dose of each ED drug to start with and work your way up if the starting dose does not provide the desire benefits. Norvir, part of HIV protease inhibitor regimens, can boost blood levels of Ed drugs by slowing down the liver's clearance of those drugs, so lower doses are needed to achieve the desired effect with the fewest side effects.

In rare instances, men taking PDE5 inhibitors have reported a sudden decrease or loss of vision. It is not possible to determine whether these events are related directly to these medicines or to other factors. If you experience sudden decrease or loss of vision, stop taking PDE5 inhibitors and call a doctor right away.

Sudden decrease or loss of hearing has been rarely reported in people taking PDE5 inhibitors. It is not possible to determine whether these events are related directly to the PDE5 inhibitors or to other factors. If you experience sudden decrease or loss of hearing, stop taking the oral ED drug and contact a doctor right away.

If you have prostate problems or high blood pressure for which you take medicines called alpha blockers, your doctor may start you on a lower dose of ED drugs.

People who use recreational drugs called "poppers" like amyl nitrite and butyl nitrite should be careful while using ED drugs since a sudden decrease in blood pressure can occur.

PERSONAL COMMENT: I have a lot of side effects on these drugs. Flushing of my face is common. Red eyes make me look like I smoked pot. Sinus congestion happens as soon as the drug enters my blood stream. And heart burn happens a few hours later. I have had a lot of lower back issues and Cialis definitely makes them worse, even at a lower daily dose. Taking over-the-counter loratadine (brand name: Claritin), ibuprofen and Propose helps me prevent the side effects, but that means that I have to take 3 extra pills with these drugs. Talk about a pill burden to get a stronger erection!

Other options for men who need an extra erectile boost while using testosterone replacement:

Yohimbine—Available over-the-counter or by prescription (Yocon); increases sex organ sensitivity. It can raise blood pressure and cause insomnia and anxiety, so talk to your doctor. A small study showed that men who used yohimbine with the amino acid arginine had better erections (read section on supplements in this book)

Muse (alprostadil)—this is a prescription pellet that inserts into the urethra to produce an erection. Not very popular since some men do not respond well or are afraid to hurt themselves if they do not stick the pellet applicator carefully through the external urethral orifice of the penis head. You can ask your urologist for a sample with a training video that comes with it to see if this option is for you.

Trimix or Quadmix—Available by prescription from compounding pharmacies. These are mixtures of prostaglandins and papaverine that increase blood flow and retention into the penis. Prostaglandins are mediators and have a variety of strong physiological effects, such as regulating the contraction and relaxation of smooth muscle tissue. Prostaglandins are not hormones and they are not produced at one discrete site, but rather in many places throughout the human body.

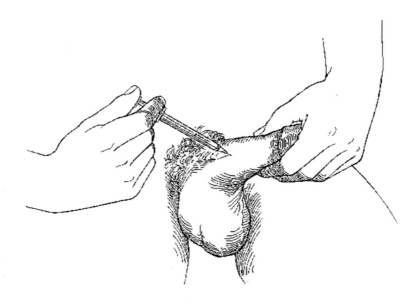

Figure 16. Injection of Trimix on the side of the penis

Trimix is a mixture of two prostaglandins (phentolamine and alprostadil) plus papaverine (a vasodilator medication) that increase blood flow to the penis and cause strong and lasting erections, with or without sexual stimulation. These compounds appear to act together to increase arterial inflow, dilate smooth muscles, and restrict venous outflow promoting erectile rigidity with greater success and in smaller doses than if these compounds were used as single therapies.

An example of a dosage combination for tri-mix is 10 micrograms of alprostadil, 500 micrograms of phentolamine and 15 mg of papaverine. Dosing of tri-mix preparations has not been standardized.

Trimix is injected directly into the side of the penis through a fine-gauge "insulin-style" needle in very small amounts (0.1-0.5 cc) that increase blood flow to the penis. It results in strong and lasting erections. The main potential side effect are hematomas (bruising), fibrosis if used too frequently and on the same injection site, pain, and dangerously long-lasting erections (priaprism). Priaprism may sound great but this can literally kill your penis by causing gangrene of the tissue after stagnant blood coagulates inside it. I know men who had to go to an emergency room 8 hours after having used too much Trimix and have the blood drained from their penis. To ensure perfect injection technique and dosing, it is imperative to be trained on how to dose this with the help of an urologist.

Compounding pharmacies sell two types of Trimix formulations: Freeze dried (powder to be mixed later with water) or pre-mixed vials. Some men find the freeze dried form not to be as effective.

It is extremely important to remember never to use Viagra, Cialis, or Levitra before or at the same time as you use Trimix. This is a dangerous combination that can increase the risk of priaprism. Be particularly careful with Cialis since it can stay in your blood stream for a longer time. I know someone who had priaprism since he had forgotten he had taken Cialis two days before using Trimix.

Most men who use Trimix love it, even if they have had to learn the hard way about priaprism during one instance. Most of these men did not respond well nor had too many side effects to oral agents like Viagra or Cialis.

For instructions on how to inject Trimix, read:

infertility-male.com/erectdys/injxn1.htm

For instructions for physicians on how to treat priaprism in the unfortunate case that it happens:

emedicine.medscape.com/article/777603-diagnosis

A 10 cc bottle of Trimix can cost from $70 to $100 in compounding pharmacies. If a dose of 0.15 cc is needed per erection, this bottle can be good for 67 erections. In comparison with Cialis and Viagra ($16 a pill), this option seems economical.

Caverject— This is an injectable form of alprostadil. Injections of alprostadil have been reported to cause pain, bleeding, hematomas and scar tissue leading to Peyronie's Disease (excessive curvature of the penis) in some patients. Caverjet is available by prescription and it is not a compounded product, so some doctors who are not comfortable prescribing compounded products feel more at ease prescribing it. However, it is not as effective as Trimix, it requires a large injection volume, and it comes preloaded in syringes with thick needles. It is also 10 times more expensive than Trimix but several insurance companies pay for it (Trimix is rarely covered by insurance). This injection into the penis that produces an erection that can last 1 to 2 hours. Follow instructions from your urologist since overdosing can also cause priaprism.

For the best treatment algorithm for physicians who want to learn more about how to prescribe, dose and manage injectable ED drugs like Trimix, Caverjet and other formulations, this article is probably the most comprehensive. It was written by Jeffrey A. Albaugh, who is an Advanced Practice Urology Clinical Nurse Specialist at Northwestern Memorial Wellness Institute in Chicago:

medscape.com/viewarticle/551563_print

Penile restriction rings—these rubber or leather restricting bands (commonly known as "cock rings") can be very effective at maintaining erections after the penis fills up with blood. Be careful not to use it too tight. Neoprene and leather rings are the most common. They can be found online.

Other options are penile vacuum devices and penile implants. Due to the scope of this book, these two options will not be reviewed. Plenty of information can be found by Googling those terms.

Erectile Dysfunction Drugs in Clinical Research

We are constantly bombarded in the media with ads of the current treatment options men have when it comes to erectile dysfunction. Viagra, Cialis and Levitra have become blockbuster medications that have been proven to be very effective for men who cannot get an erection on their own. Some drugs in development are aiming at causing fewer side effects or actually increasing sexual desire (with the current oral drugs, you still need to be aroused for them to work).

It is estimated that some degree of ED affects half of all men over the age of 40 and that 150 million men worldwide suffer from ED. Up to 35% of men with ED are non-responsive to standard therapies with phosphodiesterase-5 inhibitors, representing an estimated market of $500 to $600 million per year. So, there is a huge interest from pharmaceutical companies to keep researching new drugs in this field.

Out of many that are being tested, there are about 4 new erectile dysfunction medications that have made it through several clinical trials and many of them are in the final stages of being approved. The ED market is an extremely competitive field. Viagra will lose its patent in 2012 and generic versions will become widely available. Whether this will mean that Viagra will be cheaper in the United States then is yet to be seen. Many drugs have become generic and yet their prices do not drop when that happens.

What products are in the ED pipeline?

Avanafil:

Being developed by Vivus, this is the one that is showing the most potential and is almost ready to hit the market. Phase 3 studies that have already been conducted that showed that Avanfil can work in as little as 15 minutes. I have not seen its safety profile. I hope it has less sinus stuffiness and flushing than the currently available ED drugs.

Zoraxel:

This medication is being developed by Rexahn Pharmaceuticals. Zoraxel so far has been proven to be very safe with limited side effects. It completed its safety and dosing studies, so it is right behind Avanafil in its development process.

Zoraxel works on areas in the brain that relate to arousal, erection and release, which may work on performance anxiety. It should be ready for sale by 2013 of no surprises arise in the studies.

Zydena (udenafil):

Made by a Korean Pharmaceutical manufacturer called Dong-A Pharmaceuticals, this medication has actually already been shown in phase 2 studies to be effective and safe. It seems to work faster than Viagra, but this claim is yet to be proven. I do not know if its side effect profile is better than the currently available oral drugs.

Although Russian and Malaysian men have access to Zydena, countries such as the US and Canada will have to wait since the approval processes in these countries go through phases and are much more detailed and complex.

Bremelanotide:

This drug is made by Palatin Technologies. It will be administered subcutaneously. It is a synthetic peptide in the class of melanocortin agonists that is a candidate for treatment of male erectile dysfunction and female sexual dysfunction (FSD).

While being studied for producing a tanning effect without the sun, the sexual enhancing actions of the peptide were discovered accidentally. It actually increases sexual arousal and desire unlike the current ED drugs that only improve erections after arousal. The manufacturer claims that bremelanotide activates the melanocortin receptors in the central nervous system that are responsible for arousal and erections.

The company had tested an oral form of the drug in previous studies, finding it very effective at increasing arousal and erectile function but with nausea as one of the side effects. The manufacturer claims that the subcutaneous formulation will have no such side effect, but it is yet to be proven in studies. I am also not sure if the drug will increase skin pigmentation in some people.

Some men are buying products similar to this one online and claim that they work well for arousal and tanning.

I will be following this field up and post any updates on testosteronewisdom.com, my blog testosteronewisdom.blogspot.com or Facebook page called "Testosterone Replacement Therapy Discussion".

Medications that could cause decreased sex drive or erectile dysfunction:

Medications can cause erectile dysfunction in some men. A great review of all studies of drugs that affect sexual function in men was provided by Dr. Walter K.H. Krause in his book "Drugs Compromising Male Sexual Health". He was able to identify evidence from different studies (many uncontrolled and small) about the common classes of prescription medications that can cause erectile dysfunction. It is not known if testosterone replacement can counteract the effects of these medication classes. Among the medications are:

- Antidepressants: Selective serotonin reuptake inhibitors (SSRIs), tricyclic antidepressants, monoamine oxidase inhibitors

- Blood pressure medications (antihypertensives): Alpha andregenergic antagonists, beta-blockers, diuretics, guanethidine, methyldopa

- Narcotics and opiates

- Barbiturates and benzodiazepines

- Hormone related products: Anabolic steroids, antiandrogens used in prostate cancer, estrogens, medroxyprogesterone, 5-alpha-reductase inhibitors (Proscar, Propecia)

- Anti-acids: Histamine 2 receptor antagonists (Tagamet), proton pump inhibitors (Prilosec)

- Cholesterol –lowering agents: Bile acid sequestrants, fenofibrates (Tricor, etc), statins (Lipitor, etc)

Fatigue

If no improvements in fatigue are observed after 6 weeks of testosterone replacement, factors beyond hypogonadism may be present.
Thyroid and adrenal function should be checked to ensure that those two glands are working properly. Sleep apnea can also be a factor involved in the failure to improve stamina. Depression may still need to be addressed with the proper medications and counseling.

Thyroid Function:
The thyroid is a butterfly-shaped endocrine gland located in the lower front of the neck. It produces thyroxine or T4, which is converted to tririodothyronine, or T3. T4 production is controlled by thyroid stimulating hormone or TSH, a hormone produced by the pituitary. Hypothyroidism, or low thyroid hormone production, can cause sexual dysfunction as well as depression, fatigue, dry skin and hair, weight gain and increased sensitivity to the cold. Blood tests to measure TSH, T4 and T3 are readily available and widely used.

The American Thyroid Association (thyroid.org) has great comprehensive information on how to determine if you have hypothyrodism that could be causing your fatigue.

Testosterone may decrease levels of thyroxin-binding globulin, resulting in decreased total T4 serum levels and increased resin uptake of T3 and T4. Free thyroid hormone levels remain unchanged, however, and there is no clinical evidence of thyroid dysfunction.

Once thyroid hormone blood levels have been normalized, testosterone tends to increase naturally.

Adrenal Function:

The adrenal glands, located in the abdomen above the kidneys, regulate stress in the human body. When the body encounters an emergency situation, the adrenal glands release hormones, such as adrenaline, that enable the body to respond accordingly. You may have encountered this reaction, called the "fight or flight" response, if you have encountered danger, fear or shock. Adrenal fatigue is the controversial idea that the adrenal glands can become worn out, creating illness, if continually over stimulated. Proponents of the "adrenal fatigue" theory hold that the adrenal glands may be over worked in some individuals and therefore become "fatigued" and unable to produce sufficient hormones.   When your adrenal glands become exhausted, your natural cortisol levels drop significantly. Cortisol is your naturally occurring stress hormone. In addition to low sex drive and infertility, symptoms of adrenal fatigue may include chronic fatigue, low blood pressure and low blood sugar, dizziness, headaches, anxiety or panic attacks, depression and other equally debilitating problems.

Some doctors may prescribe low doses of corticoid steroids if your morning levels of cortisol (measure by blood, saliva or urine tests) are low. But be careful with corticoid steroids since they can increase fat mass and decrease bone density if given in doses that exceed what the healthy adrenals would produce.

DHEA:

The adrenal glands also produce dihydroepiandrosterone (DHEA), the most abundant hormone found in the blood stream. The body uses DHEA as the starting material for producing the sex hormones testosterone and estrogen in men. Studies have shown that it only increases testosterone in women. The production of DHEA diminishes in most people after age 40. In people aged 70 years, DHEA levels will be approximately 30 percent lower than what they were at age 25. Low blood levels of DHEA have been associated with many degenerative conditions.

Some controversial and non-conclusive studies have shown that people with immune deficiencies and fatigue may benefit from supplementation with this hormone. It is still available over-the-counter in the United States. This may change soon due to a new bill passed by Congress that classifies it as a performance-enhancing steroid (no studies have shown that it has such effect).

One study showed that women with the correct levels of DHEA can convert it into testosterone as their body needs while men do not benefit to the same degree. You need a blood test to know if you have low DHEA-S since most of the DHEA converts into this sulfated form. Common doses for women are 5 to 30 mg a day, while men tend to benefit from 25-100 mg per day (to bring low levels of DHEA-S to normal)

All the hormones mentioned can be tested with blood tests or by using the easy-do-it-at-home mail order saliva hormone tests that are available without a prescription. Mail-order saliva tests for testosterone, DHEA-S, estradiol, and cortisol are offered by Great Smokies Laboratory at 1-800-522-4762.

NOTE: Do not use DHEA supplements unless your blood levels of DHEA-S are low. If low, start at a low dose and get your DHEA-S tested again after a month. Men who use DHEA supplements may have problems with higher estrogen levels since DHEA can also metabolize into estradiol. This could result in gynecomastia and water retention. If you start taking DHEA, have your blood levels checked to make sure they are not above normal. There are many claims about DHEA being an anti-aging and an anti-cancer cure, but none of these claims has been substantiated with strong data.

Sleep Apnea:
Sleep apnea is a sleep disorder in which a person briefly stops breathing or breathes shallowly many times during sleep and therefore does not get enough restful sleep; oxygen levels drop in the blood, starving the brain of oxygen. In addition to causing daytime fatigue, it can increase blood pressure and cardiovascular risks. Testosterone replacement therapy has been associated with exacerbation of sleep apnea or with the development of sleep apnea, generally in men who use higher doses of testosterone or who have other identifiable risk factors for sleep apnea (high body weight, thick necks, snoring, alcohol consumption, and others). Upper-airway narrowing does not seem to be caused by testosterone replacement therapy, suggesting that testosterone replacement contributes to sleep-disordered breathing by central mechanisms rather than by means of anatomical changes in the airway.

If your spouse or partner complains that you snore loudly at night and you suffer from fatigue, tell your doctor. The only real way to find out if you have sleep apnea is to have your doctor refer you to a sleep lab for a sleep study. If you are diagnosed with sleep apnea, a **Continuous Pressure Airway Pressure (CPAP) machine** can be prescribed to help you open up your airways with a small air pump while you sleep. Some people love it while some hate wearing a mask while being hooked up to a machine at night. I have seen men regain their quality of life after starting

CPAP. It is paid by insurance, Medicare and most HMOs.

A new emerging option for those who hate CPAP machines with mild to moderate apnea is the use of **oral appliance**. Worn in the mouth like an orthodontic appliance during sleep, oral appliances keep the soft tissue from collapsing and interrupting normal breathing patterns. The purpose of the oral appliance may be to reposition the lower jaw, tongue, soft palate, and hyoid bone into a certain position, to keep the airway open with stabilization of the tongue and jaw, or to provide artificial muscle tone to prevent collapse and resulting airway blockage. The doctors will fit your oral appliance for comfort by using a mold of your mouth to design your unique fit.

Sleep apnea appliances fall into two categories: fixed and adjustable. Here are brief descriptions of some commonly used sleep apnea dental appliances:

TAP® 3 (Thornton Adjustable Positioner)

The TAP® 3 is the smallest, most comfortable member of the TAP family. It is a two-part custom-created sleep apnea appliance that fits over the teeth in much the same way as a sports mouth guard. The TAP® 3 projects the jaw forward to prevent the tongue and soft tissues from impeding the airway. The lower jaw positioner is adjustable, which means that it can be altered to suit the comfort level of the wearer. The TAP® 3 appliance can accommodate the three main types of malocclusion, and allows the lips to fully close.

OASYS Appliance

The OASYS appliance is designed to move the base of the tongue toward the front of the mouth by gently repositioning the jawbone (mandible). This shift opens the oropharynx and strengthens the upper airway. An extension of the upper shield projects toward the nose, creating a larger nasal opening and less resistance to normal airflow. This adjustable appliance is comfortable to wear and extremely patient friendly.

Klearway™ Appliance

The Klearway™ Appliance is generally used to alleviate obstructive sleep disorder and eliminate snoring. The patient or dentist can project the jaw forwards in increments of .25mm at a time. This ensures maximum comfort for the sleeper. The Klearway™ appliance is made from Variflex™ heat softening acrylic, which makes it easier to insert. Running warm water over the appliance makes it pliable, but once placed in the desired position, the acrylic hardens again.

Herbst Telescopic Appliance

The Herbst appliance is held in the mouth by clasps and friction grips. It is made of acrylic, and contains adjustable metal wiring. The advantage of this appliance is that the wearer is able to move vertically and laterally without dislodging the appliance. The Herbst appliance is usually used in mild and moderate cases of sleep apnea, and can also alleviate loud snoring effectively.

If you have questions or concerns about sleep apnea appliances, please ask your dentist. To locate a dentist in your area that uses these products, visit:

endsnore.com/request-form.aspx

Stimulants:

Some physicians prescribe drugs like Nuvigil, Ritalin or Adderall when everything else fails.

Armodafinil (brand name Nuvigil) is used to treat excessive sleepiness caused by narcolepsy (a condition of excessive daytime sleepiness) or shift work sleep disorder (sleepiness during scheduled waking hours and difficulty falling asleep or staying asleep during scheduled sleeping hours in people who work at night or on rotating shifts). Armodafinil is also used along with breathing devices or other treatments to prevent excessive sleepiness caused by obstructive sleep apnea/hypopnea syndrome. Armodafinil is in a class of medications called wakefulness-promoting agents. It works by changing the amounts of certain natural substances in the area of the brain that controls sleep and wakefulness. Some insurance companies do not want to pay for it. It is not an amphetamine and it does not require a special prescription since it not a class III DEA regulated drug. Many doctors have samples so that you can try it before you commit to using it.

Ritalin and Adderall (both come in cheaper generics) are also being prescribed to people with severe fatigue that does not respond to usual means.

Methylphenidate (Ritalin, Ritalin SR, Methylin, Methylin ER) is used as part of a treatment program to control symptoms of attention deficit hyperactivity disorder (ADHD) in adults and children. Methylphenidate is also used to treat narcolepsy. Methylphenidate is in a class of medications called central nervous system (CNS) stimulants. It works by changing the amounts of certain natural substances in the brain.

Adderall is a brand-name psychostimulant medication composed of racemic amphetamine aspartate monohydrate, racemic amphetamine sulfate, dextroamphetamine saccharide and dextroamphetamine sulfate, which is thought to work by increasing the amount of dopamine and norepinephrine in the brain. Adderall is widely reported to increase alertness, libido, concentration and overall cognitive performance while decreasing user fatigue. It is available in two formulations: IR (**I**nstant **R**elease) and XR (e**X**tended **R**elease). The immediate release formulation is indicated for use in Attention Deficit Hyperactivity Disorder (ADHD) and narcolepsy, while the XR formulation is approved for use only with ADHD. In the United States, Adderall is a Schedule II drug under the Controlled Substance Act due to having significant abuse and addiction potential. It requires a triplicate prescription in many states.

There is some concerning data on the use of stimulants and increased cardiovascular risks, so it is important to talk to your doctor about this. Sometimes calculated risks are taken when nothing else works to regain a normal quality of life!

If you and your doctor decide that stimulants are a reasonable option, you will need to review the many potential drug interactions, physical health and mental health complications that can occur.

Over-the-Counter Supplement: SAMe
SAMe (SAM-e, S-adenosyl-methionine, or S-adenosyl-L-methionine) is a naturally occurring compound that is found in every cell in the body. It is produced within the body from the essential sulfur-containing amino acid methionine. Protein-rich foods are sources of this amino acid. It is an antioxidant and it has shown to have liver protecting properties.

SAMe is generally considered safe when taken in appropriate doses. People with bipolar (manic/depressive) disorder should be aware that it could trigger a manic phase. People taking standard antidepressants, including MAO inhibitors, SSRIs, and tricyclics should not take SAMe except on a physician's advice. It has been shown to help SSRI drugs work better when used in combination. It is fairly well tolerated but be it can cause jitteriness or gut problems in some.

I am convinced that this supplement works for depression and fatigue. I have taken 400 mg twice a day for a few months and can definitely feel a difference. I actually get reminded when I do not take it by my having decreased energy. An added bonus is that it can also decrease liver enzymes.

SAMe is not cheap. There are many different manufacturers but I use the Jarrow Formulas brand, as I trust their quality control. It comes in foil-protected 200 mg-capsules since it tends to lose its effectiveness when exposed to air.

Here is a summary of studies that show that it works as well as commonly prescribed antidepressants, and also some data on liver function and arthritis pain:

healthyplace.com/Communities/Depression/treatment/alternative/ sam-e.asp

I am also including a study done at ACRIA that also found benefits in treating depression in people living with HIV:

pubmedcentral.nih.gov/articlerender.fcgi?artid=535560

Talk to your doctor before taking this supplement. Do not stop taking your antidepressants to switch to SAMe since it has not been fully studied in large controlled studies.

Start at a small dose of 100 mg twice a day on an empty stomach and see how you feel with that dose. If you do not feel any more energy, increase the dose to 200 mg twice a day and so on until the maximum dose of 400 mg twice is achieved. You may have to lower the dose if your start feeling anxious.

PERSONAL COMMENTS: Because of terrible bouts with fatigue in the past, I was referred to a sleep lab and diagnosed with mild sleep apnea. I tried CPAP with different masks (they are smaller ones with "nose pillows" and many other designs, so don't give up early without trying different styles). I could not get used to it. I have had my thyroid and adrenal functions checked without finding any problems. I have tried Nuvigil, Adderall, and SAMe with good results for my fatigue. Unfortunately I get anxious if I use them for long periods, so I only use them as needed. What has made the most difference, besides keeping my testosterone in the upper side of the normal range, is going to bed around the same time at night and waking up also at the same time. Traveling and other factors can interfere with maintaining a normal sleep cycle, but the fact is I need to listen to my body's needs. I can usually be tired enough to get better sleep by the time bedtime arrives if I avoid caffeine after 3 pm and don't exercise too late at night. Being aware of any potential bouts of depression and negative thinking has also helped me to be proactive about not letting my energy levels plummet.

-6-

Supplements

Supplements That Claim to Improve Sexual Function and/or Testosterone

Many people either don't trust big drug companies or they prefer the idea of using products that they see as "natural" or "herbal". Therefore I'm going to address a few of these. Please keep in mind a general rule about supplements: They are not regulated by the FDA. Most companies make a lot of unsubstantiated claims as long as they have a tiny sentence on their label that says "this statement has not been reviewed by the FDA". Lack of regulation leads to a wide range in potency of the product between manufacturers (one reason it can make some studies hard to verify). I have always turned to the people at the non-profit organizations the Houston Buyers Club or the New York Buyers Club for assistance in choosing my supplements. ConsumerLabs.org is also a good resource since they test supplements to determine who is lying about their ingredients, but you need to have a paid subscription to the site.

Testosterone prohormones such as androstenedione, androstenediol, and dehydroepiandrosterone (DHEA) have been heavily marketed as testosterone-enhancing and muscle-building nutritional supplements for the past decade. Concerns over the safety of prohormone supplement use prompted the United States Food and Drug Administration to call for a ban on androstenedione sales, and Congress passed the Anabolic Steroid Control Act of 2004, which classifies androstenedione and 17 other steroids as controlled substances. As of January 2005, these substances cannot be sold without prescription. Contrary to marketing claims, research to date indicates that the use of prohormone nutritional supplements (DHEA, androstenedione, androstenediol, and other steroid hormone supplements) does not produce either anabolic or ergogenic effects in men.

Korean red ginseng

Two double-blind, placebo-controlled trials, involving a total of about 135 people found evidence that Korean red ginseng may improve erectile function when compared with placebo. A dose of 900 mg was given three times daily and the study period was 8 weeks.

In an analysis combining the results of six controlled trials, researchers found some evidence supporting the benefits of Korean red ginseng. There are doubts about this conclusion as these studies were small size and non-validated.

L-arginine

L-arginine is an amino acid with many functions in the body. One of these is its role in the production of nitric oxide which helps relax blood vessels. This relaxation is essential in the development of an erection. Drugs like Viagra increase the body's sensitivity to the natural rise in nitric oxide that occurs when we get sexually excited. Another approach might be to raise nitric oxide levels, which led to the idea of trying L-arginine.

Oral arginine supplements may increase nitric oxide levels in the penis and elsewhere. The main data that generated some interest in the use of arginine for erectile dysfunction came from a small double-blind trial in which 50 men with erectile dysfunction received either 5 g of L-arginine or placebo daily for six weeks (**NOTE**: a capsule contains 500 mg, so 10 capsules a day!). More men in the treated group experienced improvement in sexual performance than in the placebo group. However, a double-blind crossover study of 32 men found no benefit with 1,500 mg of arginine given daily for 17 days. The significant difference in dose and shorter course of treatment may explain the discrepancy between these two trials.

L-arginine has been advertised as "natural Viagra" but there is little evidence that it works. Drugs based on raising nitric oxide levels in the penis have not worked out for pharmaceutical developers; the body seems to adjust to the higher levels and maintain the same level of response.

Arginine supplementation appears to work only in those whose erectile dysfunction is due to low nitric oxide levels. In other words, arginine would be unlikely to help those whose decreased libido is due to factors other than low NO levels. Remember, erectile dysfunction is a complex syndrome and may be due to many different factors, both chemical and psychological.

NOTE: Large doses of L-arginine can activate the herpes virus in those who have been exposed to it. You may want to take medication for herpes treatment if you decide to use this supplement. L-arginine is also commonly used in bodybuilding supplements since it can cause transient increases in growth hormone.

Yohimbine and yohimbe

Yohimbine HCl is an indole alkaloid found in the bark of the *Pausinystalia yohimbe* tree. Yohimbe bark has been used in Africa for centuries as an aphrodisiac. It is available as a supplement but is also available by prescription in the United States under the trade-name Yocon. It too helps with erections by relaxing blood vessels in the penis.

Yohimbine has been studied in combination with L-arginine. One study of 45 men found that one-time use of this combination therapy an hour or two before intercourse improved erectile function in those with only moderate erectile dysfunction. Arginine and yohimbine were both taken at a dose of 6 g, which would require a lot of capsules (if taken in powder form a tea spoon has 5 g). All the related studies were very small. I doubt that there are future larger studies planned since we now have effective erectile dysfunction drugs that work.

NOTE: Yohimbine (and yohimbe) present a number of safety risks related to increased heart rate, blood pressure, insomnia, anxiety, and liver/kidney dysfunction. It is best to use this under physician supervision.

PERSONAL COMMENT: I have taken Yocon and found it too "speedy" for me.

Carnitine

Carnitine is a compound that helps transport fatty acids for the generation of metabolic energy. In addition to its apparent benefit for diabetes, the heart and affecting bone mass it may have benefit with erectile dysfunction. Propionyl-l-carnitine at 2 g/day plus acetyl-l-carnitine also at 2 g/day and testosterone (testosterone undecanoate 160 mg/week) were separately compared with placebo. The results indicated that both carnitine and testosterone improved erectile function; however, while testosterone significantly increased prostate volume, carnitine did not. Other studies seem to indicate that propionyl-l-carnitine at 2 g/day enhanced the effectiveness of sildenafil (Viagra) in a small group of men with diabetes who were not responding to sildenafil on at least eight occasions.

PERSONAL COMMENT: I have taken these two forms of carnitine and can honestly say that I have not felt any difference in the erectile department. I take the supplement daily for lipid control and support of my mitochondria, however.

Zinc

Zinc is a trace mineral that is second only to iron in the body. Zinc is involved in many physiological processes in the body such as wound repair, proper functioning of the immune system, cell division, cell growth, proper taste and smell sensation. This important mineral also plays a role in the proper metabolism of carbohydrates and for normal childhood growth and sexual development. Men who are deficient in zinc may have an issue with fertility and libido, while women who are deficient in zinc may have an upset menstrual cycle.

Severe zinc deficiency is known to negatively affect sexual function. Since marginal zinc deficiency is relatively common, it is logical to suppose that supplementation with zinc may be helpful for some men. This hypothesis has only been studied in men receiving kidney dialysis but the results were promising. You can take too much zinc, so check with your doctor about how much is enough.

NOTE: I take 50 mg of zinc plus 3 mg of copper a day to support my immune system. Zinc can lower copper, which is also important for the immune system. I take a product made by Jarrow that combines the two. But zinc does not increase testosterone, but can help support testosterone production.

Maca

The herb maca (Lepidium meyenii) is another supplement advertised as "herbal Viagra." In one study of rats, maca enhanced male sexual function. For those of you who aren't rats, there is one published human trial. In this small, 12-week, double-blind, placebo-controlled study, use of maca at 1,500 mg or 3,000 mg increased male sexual desire but no data was shown on the quality of erections. The claims that it increases testosterone have not been substantiated with data.

Tribulus Terrestris

Tribulus terrestris L. (Zygophyllaceae) have been used as an aphrodisiac both in the Indian and Chinese traditional systems of medicine. Administration of *Tribulus terrestris* extract (TT) increased sexual behavior and intracavernous pressure both in normal and castrated rats and these effects were probably due to the androgen increasing property of TT

In a study done in Bulgaria, twenty-one healthy young 20–36 years old men were randomly separated into three groups—two experimental (each $n = 7$) and a control (placebo) one ($n = 7$). The experimental groups were named TT1 and TT2 and the subjects were assigned to consume 20 and 10 mg/kg body weight per day of *Tribulus terrestris* extract, respectively, separated into three daily intakes for 4 weeks. No changes in testosterone, androstenedione and luteinizing hormone blood levels were observed with either dose.

Other Herbs

There are other herbs that have been promoted as improving sexual function in men. Among these are Ashwagandha, Avena sativa (oat straw), eleutherococcus (the so-called Siberian ginseng), L-citrulline, *Macuna pruriens*, molybdenum, muira puama or potency wood (you have to love the name), pygeum, *Polypodium vulgare*, Rhodi-ola rosea, saw palmetto, schisandra, suma, traditional Chinese herbal medicine, and deer or antelope velvet antle. There are no well-designed, controlled scientific studies that support any of those claims.

Many herbal supplements that claim to improve sexual function have been found to contain Viagra or Cialis purchased in China at cheaper prices. The FDA has stopped those companies from selling them but many keep reappearing in the unregulated supplement market.

All supplements that actually increase testosterone, such as androstenedione, are considered performance-enhancing drugs. They have been banned in the United States. This is just as well as they only increased testosterone for a few hours and had the potential to cause liver problems. New supplements keep appearing on the market and claim to increase the body's production of testosterone or growth hormone. Be very skeptical about those claims and do not waste your money on them!

The best and safest way to supplement your testosterone is to *use approved products under your physician's supervision and care.*

-7-

Miscellaneous Health Tips to Support Healthy Testosterone

Testosterone therapy can be of tremendous benefit in restoring your energy and sense of well-being but you shouldn't rely on hormone replacement as being the only change that you make in your health regimen. Better health involves some important lifestyle choices. I've also included other tips based on my own experiences.

Tips for Maximizing Your Health and Response to Testosterone Replacement Therapy

- Exercise with weights/machines three to four times a week for no more than one hour; this helps build muscle. On alternate days do cardiovascular exercise (elliptical trainer, fast walking, light jogging, etc.) for at least 30 minutes a day; this helps with stamina and overall health. Make sure that you sweat! Discuss your exercise program with your doctor before you start.

- At the start of any exercise program and every three months measure your chest, thighs, arms, and abdomen. Weigh yourself weekly.

- It is not a bad idea if you are over 40 to ask your doctor for a full body DEXA (dual X Ray Absorptiometry) scan so that you can know how many grams of muscle, fat and bone you have in every part of your body, and then repeat every three years to monitor changes. Sometimes it is difficult to find a radiology clinic that does full body DEXAs since they are usually accustomed to doing only DEXA's of the hips or spine area for post menopausal women with bone loss.

- Take at least a multivitamin a day with meals. I like the Energy Pack from Super Nutrition.

- Motivate yourself with a buddy or support system. I don't mean just for exercise either; surround yourself with some wise and upbeat people.

- If you have to use stimulants, such as coffee and green tea, use them only in moderation. I personally love a cup of espresso 30 minutes before a work out.

- Get good quality sleep. Talk with your doctor if you're not getting it. Refer to the section on fatigue in this book.

- Manage stress with relaxation techniques and hobbies. Learn to let go of anger and unrealistic expectations.

- Get at least 20 minutes a day of sunshine (avoid the face to prevent wrinkles). Your body needs it to make vitamin D for bone health. Get your vitamin D blood levels checked and supplement at with at least 2000 IU per day if found to have low blood levels (ask your doctor about this test).

- Sweat. Use a pedometer or download a pedometer app in your phone to try to walk at least 10,000 steps a day. Increase your cardio by parking far, taking the stairs, walking the dog, or dancing. Make it fun!

- Choose your supplements wisely. Beware of companies claiming that their "growth hormone or testosterone precursors" work; they don't. Most weight loss supplements have stimulants that can affect mood and increase blood pressure and cardiovascular risks.

- Treat depression quickly with exercise, therapy, antidepressants, and a good support system.

- Get a Pneumovax vaccine every five years. Pneumovax is a vaccine against bacterial pneumonia.

- If you've never had hepatitis A or B, ask your doctor about getting vaccinated against them.

How to Protect Your Heart

- Do not smoke!

- Manage stress and keep your blood pressure in check.

- Decrease high triglycerides with Omega 3 fatty acids (cold water fish oils) and by cutting down on sugars. The American Heart Association (AHA) recommends at least two 3 oz servings of fish

per week. Some experts recommend eating four 3-ounce servings
of fatty fish per week for people with heart disease or cardiac risk
factors. The following have higher levels of omega-3 fatty acids:

- o   Anchovies
- o   Bluefish
- o   Carp
- o   Catfish
- o   Halibut
- o   Herring
- o   Lake trout
- o   Mackerel
- o   Pompano
- o   Salmon
- o   Tuna

• Improve fat utilization and energy with 2 to 4 grams a day of over-
the-counter L-Carnitine (prescription Carnitor).

• Increase your HDL (the good cholesterol) if it's low with Niacin
at 500-1500 per day. Start with lower dose to minimize "flushing"
and take an aspirin 20 min before (Niaspan is the prescription
grade). I have never been able to take it for too long without
having that horrible flushing feeling, however.

• Maximize soluble and insoluble fiber (see below).

• If everything else fails to lower your cholesterol and triglycerides,
use prescription lipid lowering agents (statins, fibrates, etc).

• If you take lipid lowering drugs, don't forget to take 300 mg a
day of Coenzyme Q10 since it has been shown to be low in those
taking those medications. This supplement can protect the heart
and muscle tissue from damage.

• Take an 81mg baby aspirin a day (with your doctor's approval).

• Go to get your teeth cleaned twice a year and floss daily. Heart
health has been linked to oral health.

Nutritional Tips:

- Shop mostly in the outer part of the grocery store where the fresh produce, meats, and milk products/eggs are.

- Do not skip breakfast (keep an eye on sugar and refined flour products!)

- Try to eat several smaller meals or snacks instead of two to three large ones.

- Eat more almonds, walnuts, pecans and pistachios (good cholesterol lowering fats).

- Eat fruits and vegetables of all colors. Each has a different antioxidant profile.

- Avoid sodas, sweet drinks and fruits juices (fruit sounds healthy but the juice part brings in too many sugars). Consuming sugar daily can affect your metabolism, create insulin resistance, make you fat, and have all kinds of negative health consequences. Watch this lecture about the damaging effects of sugar and fructose: http://www.youtube.com/watch?v=dBnniua6-oM

- Drink lots of water.

- Eat a high protein, complex carbohydrate- rich meal after work outs.

- Manage your intake of caffeine (it reduces appetite but can increase anxiety). Do not have any caffeine after 4 pm

- Get a slow cooker so that you come back from work to a warm meal. They come with great cook books.

- Cook for the week and freeze in individual serving sized containers.

- Reduce saturated (animal) fats, fried foods and hydrogenated oils to a minimum

- Use good fats: olive oil, nuts, and avocados.

- Minimize hidden sugars like fructose (sweets, sodas, and many processed foods are high in fructose corn syrup). Read the labels of food you buy.

- Eat adequate amounts (0.7-1 gm/lb/day) of protein (fish, eggs, cottage cheese, lean meats, chicken, whey, yogurt, nuts, etc).

- Eat more high-fiber, nutrient and fluid-rich, low calorie, low glycemic carbs like: Oatmeal, multi-grain breads, vegetables, fruits, roots, greens, wild rice and beans. If you do not consume at least 20 grams of fiber a day, supplement with supplements like Citrucell or Benefiber purchased in any grocery store.

- Healthy grocery shopping list:
    o Mix of almonds and other nuts
    o Beans and other legumes (you can buy frozen ones)
    o Spinach and other green leafy vegetables
    o Broccoli and cabbage
    o Low fat dairy, yogurt (Greek style, no sugar added)
    o Hummus
    o Whey protein (I like the Isopure brand since it does not give me gut problems and it is very light)
    o Oatmeal (not the little packets; those are loaded with sugars)
    o Eggs (free range or Omega 3 enriched if possible)
    o Lean meats
    o Salmon, sardines and tuna
    o Whole grain breads and pasta
    o Peanut, almond, and cashew butters without hydrogenated oil (the healthy nut butters show oil and butter separated since the lack of hydrogenated oils prevents emulsification)
    o Olive oil and avocados
    o Raspberries and all berries. Whole fruits (remember no juices). You can buy frozen ones and add to whey protein shakes
    o Occasional glass of red wine per day (optional)
    o Pumpkin and sunflower seeds
    o Sweet potatoes and wild rice (the darker the rice, the

better)
- o Benefiber
- o Green tea
- o Reduced fat milk (if you are not lactose intolerant)

General Exercise Suggestions:

There is controversy in the literature about the effects of exercise on testosterone blood levels. Conflicting results may be explained by differences in the intensity and duration of the activity and the physical characteristics of the individual (e.g. age and fitness level).

Relatively short duration intense activity may lead to transient increases in testosterone concentrations. Athletes who train intensively may experience reductions in testosterone levels but not below normal clinical range. This is not necessarily a consistent phenomenon.

The important thing to remember is that when done correctly, exercise can have the following proven benefits that go beyond just looking good:

- Improved muscle function and strength.

- Reduced trunk (belly) fat

- Increased muscle mass

- Decreased LDL (bad cholesterol).

- Decreased triglycerides. Muscle hypertrophy (enlargement) induced by resistance training, may decrease triglycerides in those with high levels.

- Improved mood and decreased stress.

- Increase bone density in men and women.
- Improved aerobic function and lung capacity.

Getting Started

There are some things to consider before you start an exercise program. Get your blood pressure, heart rate, weight, body dimensions, fasting cholesterol, triglycerides, and blood sugar measured. Your doctor should be able to advise you if you are capable of exercising without health risks.

If you feel too tired and weak, start by walking every day to your best ability. Walking can increase your energy levels so you can start a more intensive exercise program as you feel better. Use a cheap pedometer to measure your daily steps; try to reach 10,000 steps a day since that amount has been associated with good cardiovascular health and fat loss.

There are two types of exercise: resistance (weight) training and cardiovascular (aerobic) exercise. Resistance training uses weights to induce muscle growth. Cardiovascular exercise improves your body's aerobic capacity (the way it uses oxygen). It also increases your metabolism so that you can burn fat, lower your bad cholesterol and triglycerides, and lower your blood sugar.

Do low-impact aerobic exercise for 20-40 minutes, three to four times a week. Exercises like walking fast, bike riding (stationary or the two-wheeler), stair stepping, and using an elliptical trainer or treadmill are all effective. Switching between different exercises can help keep your interest going. Be careful about aerobic exercise if you are losing weight involuntarily, if you are overly tired or recovering from illness.

Recommendations

Train with weights and machines three times a week for no more than one hour. Starting with machines is the safest way until you get familiar with the exercises. As you feel more confident and strong, bring in free weight exercise (hopefully with the help of a workout buddy). As you get stronger, increase your weights in every exercise. Exercise one body part per week, and do three exercises per body part. One light warm-up set and two heavier sets of eight to ten repetitions to momentary muscle failure (until you cannot do another rep) are enough for each exercise. If you do not have access to a gym, do push-ups on the floor and squats holding books or large bottles full of water at home. As long as you are "resisting" your own body weight, you are doing resistance exercise. You can also get an exercise ball and follow this great home-based workout:
myfit.ca/exercisedatabase/search.asp?muscle=Home&equipment=yes

For examples of other exercises you can do at home, visit:

weboflife.nasa.gov/exerciseandaging/chapter4_strength.html

For great resistance exercises at the gym, visit:

myfit.ca/exercisedatabase/weight_lifting_exercises.asp

Important Things to Remember

- Learn how to do each exercise correctly. Concentrate on using strict form to get the most out of each exercise and to prevent injuries.

- Make sure your muscles are warm before targeting them with more challenging weights. Warm them up with a light, high-repetition exercise set.

- Don't use your body to add momentum; cheating this way takes work away from the targeted muscles. Use a deliberate speed to increase the effectiveness of the movement.

- Use a full range of motion on all exercises. Feel the muscle stretch at the bottom and go for a momentary peak contraction at the top. Don't go too fast!

- Warm up before you work out and stretch afterwards to prevent injury. Briefly stretch the major muscle groups before your training. This helps flexibility and muscle recovery. For stretching routines, go to:_weboflife.nasa.gov/exerciseandaging/chapter4_ stretching.html

- Feel the muscles working by keeping your head in what you're doing. Focus on your muscles contracting and relaxing. Concentrate on your body exercising, not on random thoughts or people around you.

- If the weight is too light (more than 12 repetitions), try using a heavier one or do the movement more slowly and really feel the contraction. You should be barely able to finish the tenth rep if your weight is the right one. Of course, as you get stronger with time, increase your weights.

- Keep rest periods to no more than about 20-30 seconds, or shorter, depending on how tired you are from your last set. This will also help to give your heart a mini-workout.

Safety First

Always remember -- safety first! If something you do in an exercise hurts, stop! Ask for help to figure out what you're doing wrong. Maybe it's improper form. If you hurt yourself, you will hinder your progress because you won't want to work out. Learn proper form! Do not exercise if you feel you are coming down with a cold.

Commit Yourself
If you can afford it, join a gym. If you spend the money, you'll be more likely to stay with it, and consistency is the key to success in any exercise program. Also, try to find someone who is enthusiastic to train with, or get a personal trainer (if you can afford one). It's easier to stay motivated when you train with someone else who has a vital interest in your mutual success. It's also safer to have someone to spot you when you lift heavy weight.

Avoid Overtraining
Working out for more than an hour can cause overtraining which can destroy your muscles and decrease your strength. Overtraining is probably the factor most ignored by exercise enthusiasts. Prolonged exercise (overtraining) may lead to suppression of testosterone levels, possibly lasting up to several days.

In order to build muscle the body has to receive a stimulus, a reason, to grow bigger (hypertrophy). It's really very simple: the body only does what it needs to do, what it is required to do. It isn't going to suddenly expand its muscle mass because it anticipates needing more muscles. But if it is challenged to move weights around, it will respond by growing.

Another way to look at it is, if you take any body builder and put him in bed for weeks at a time, he'll begin to rapidly lose muscle mass because the body will sense that it doesn't need the extra muscle any more. By lifting weights one delivers the needed stimulus to begin muscular hypertrophy.

However, overdoing exercise stresses out the body and actually initiates the process of breaking down muscle mass as the body begins to burn its own muscles to use for fuel. This overtraining is why so many people don't grow at a satisfying rate. Even worse, these same people often will think they aren't training hard enough. They *increase* their exercise routines, thinking they just need more stimuli! And this is where the biggest error is made -- more is *not* necessarily better! It seems paradoxical that you could work out *less* and grow *more*, but this is very often the case.

Any exercise beyond that which is the exact amount of stimulus necessary to induce optimal muscle growth is called overtraining. I know this sounds non-specific but the idea is that it will vary from person to person. You need to listen to your body.

A Workout Log Is Recommended

The best reason to keep track of your workouts is so that you can see graphically what you are accomplishing. You will be able to see whether you're gaining strength at a reasonable rate. You can also analyze your pattern to see if you're overtraining. You will find when you log your workouts, that if you are overtraining, you won't be gaining in strength or muscle size. Document your workouts by keeping track of the weight you lift and the amount of reps you lift for each exercise. Then when you go in to train again the next week, you'll know what you are trying to improve upon. If you find out that you're weaker than you were the time before, and everything else like nutrition, etc. is in line, you may be training too often. For downloading workout logs, visit: www.exrx.net/WeightTraining/WorkoutLogs.html

Food and Hydration

Drink at least eight glasses of water a day to keep hydrated. Dehydration can rob you of energy for your workouts. Drink plenty of water while working out. Avoid sugary drinks, since they will cause fatigue after an initial burst of energy. Some people like to drink green tea or creatine supplements in water before a workout to help increase energy levels through a workout.

A light carbohydrate meal (fruits, carbohydrate drinks, etc.) before a workout and a protein-rich one afterwards is advisable. Keep yourself well hydrated with plenty of water throughout the workout. And get plenty of rest afterwards.

Do not work out right after eating a regular meal; wait at least two hours. If you need a snack, have some fruit and a slice of toast with peanut butter one hour or more before working out. Do not consume protein shakes before working out (leave them for after the workout). Digestion will slow down your workouts and bring your energy down. Within 30-60 minutes after the workout, feed your muscles with a balanced meal containing protein, good fats (olive oil, flaxseed oil), and complex carbohydrates, like fruits and whole grains.

Supplements like glutamine, creatine, and whey protein may be a good thing to consider. A shake containing one heaping tablespoon of glutamine, two tablespoons of Omega 3 oils, one or two scoops of whey protein, some fruit, and milk (if you are lactose intolerant try almond or rice milk, though not soy, since it may increase estrogen in both men and women), provides a good balanced meal after a workout.

Home Based Economical Exercise Helpers
I love the following three cheap devices:

1- An exercise (medicine) ball and elastic bands. You can get one at $14 at Target or any retail store. Make sure it comes with its own pump
You can use these work outs:
www.myfit.ca/exercisedatabase/search.asp?muscle=Ball&equipment=yes

2- I love the chin-up (pull-up) bars that you can install on door frames. Here is one that you do not have to install and you can move around:
www.amazon.com/Creative-Fitness-DG-Door-Gym/dp/B00029A7C0

3- Get yourself a cheap pedometer in any store to make sure you wear it from the moment you wake up until you go to bed. Ensure that you reach close to 10,000 steps a day for best aerobic capacity. I like the Omron-HJ-150-Hip-pedometer available at amazon.com

Exercise Resources
Two of the best websites for video clips of exercises and an explanation of anatomy are: www.exrx.net/Lists/Directory.html and www.myfit.ca
Also, several exercise routines are provided on our website www.medibolics.com/exercise.html
You can also find most exercise routines explained in videos on youtube. com and menshealth.com

Testosterone Replacement, Side Effects and Management

Interview With
Dr. Michael Scally

Nelson Vergel (NV): Dr. Michael Scally is a well-known expert on men's health in general, and specifically he's an expert on hormone therapy and issues surrounding testosterone replacement. Dr. Scally, can you tell us a little bit about your background?

Michael Scally (MS): My education includes a double degree major in chemistry (1975) and life sciences (1975) from the Massachusetts Institute of Technology (MIT) Cambridge, MA. From 1975 to 1980, in the MIT division of Brain Sciences & Neuroendocrinology, I researched and published investigations on neurotransmitter relationships. During this time, I entered the prestigious Health Sciences & Technology Program, a collaboration of the MIT and Harvard Medical School. In 1980, I was awarded by Harvard Medical School a Doctorate of Medicine, MD. In 1983, I completed a fellowship in anesthesiology at Parkland Southwest Memorial, in Dallas. From 1983 to 1994, I was a private practice anesthesiologist. In 1984, I set up the first ambulatory, outpatient, surgery center at Houston.

In 1994, I became interested in general and preventative medicine with a focus on endocrinology. I have been active in this area since that time.

In 1995, I inquired to Wyeth Pharmaceuticals about the association between primary pulmonary hypertension and pondimin (fenfluramine). I came to learn, this inquiry later was used as evidence in the class-action suit against Wyeth and was instrumental in showing that the known adverse effects were known to Wyeth but not revealed to the public.

During 1994, I competed in the Mr. Texas Bodybuilding Championship, placing second. While exercising, I was approached by a number of weightlifters on the medical treatment to restore the hypothalamic-pituitary axis (HPTA) after stopping anabolic steroids (AAS). Many of these same individuals also used over-the-counter (OTC) supplements.

As you might know, many bodybuilders are trying to decrease their body fat and increase their muscle mass as much as they can. And with these two specific goals in their mind, they were having a hard time because they were taking this over-the-counter supplement. Within a short time later, I discovered an over-the-counter weight loss supplement containing an ingredient, tiratricol, toxic to the thyroid. The reporting of this to the federal agency, MedWatch, was instrumental in the nationwide seizure of the supplement thus avoiding a disaster to the public health and welfare. We published our findings in the peer-reviewed literature, being the first to do so.

This spurred on my interest in the field of men's health, particularly in the field of testosterone and anabolic steroids. I recognized the use of a treatment for stopping anabolic steroids, both prescription and nonprescription, was without any scientific support. The accepted standard of care within the medical community for anabolic steroid-induced hypogonadism is to do nothing with the expectation the individual will return to normal unassisted. This is proving not to be the case and now jeopardizes the health and welfare of countless individuals.

I developed a treatment for anabolic steroid-induced hypogonadism that has been published and presented before the Endocrine Society, the American Association of Clinical Endocrinologists, American College of Sports Medicine, and the International Workshop on Adverse Drug Reactions and Lipodystrophy in HIV. The condition of anabolic steroid-induced hypogonadism is found in nonprescription and prescription AAS alike. The failure of the medical community to recognize the importance of anabolic steroid-induced hypogonadism, particularly in the research setting, is the focus of my recently published book, "Anabolic Steroids—A Question of Muscle: Human Subject Abuses in Anabolic Steroid Research."

NV: There are lots of misconceptions when it comes to testosterone replacement in men. Will you tell us, in your opinion, what are the

main misconceptions? For instance, some doctors may think that giving testosterone to somebody with low testosterone may affect the liver, or may cause cancer of the liver or prostate.

MS: There are many misconceptions regarding anabolic steroids, which include testosterone. You mentioned two of the areas: liver and prostate cancer. Other areas are enlargement of the prostate or benign prostate hypertrophy, anabolic steroid dependency, cardiovascular disease, and addiction.

I believe that many of the misconceptions come about by the politicization of anabolic steroids. As far as prescribed medicines are concerned, anabolic steroids are the only group of drugs with a law specifically aimed at their use. This has led to a lack or absence of good research. Instead, what the medical community has relied on are anecdotal and inflammatory reports.

This is probably most evident in the medical community's steadfast refusal to accept that anabolic steroids increase muscle mass and strength. We now know that anabolic steroids conclusively do increase muscle mass and strength and athletic performance.

As far as liver effects, use of the oral anabolic steroids has been reported to cause liver dysfunction and cancer. These reports are primarily in individuals with a preexisting condition treated for extended periods. The intramuscular injections and transdermal preparations do not appear to be associated with liver problems, and routine monitoring is therefore unnecessary. In the thousands of patients I have treated with testosterone, I never even think about liver problems being a contraindication, because they just do not come up.

In non-obstructive benign prostatic hyperplasia (BPH), testosterone replacement therapy is not a concern. The prostate volumes increase in an inconsistent manner. As with any treatment, careful monitoring will alert one to a problem.

As far as prostatic cancer, there is no association. In 2004, a *New England Journal of Medicine* article review of over 60 studies on testosterone replacement therapy concluded that there is no causal or association with prostate cancer.

NV: But testosterone replacement seems to be getting more and more mainstream. Ever since the introduction of gels like Androgel and Testim, more and more doctors feel comfortable prescribing testosterone. But yet, there are still a lot of fears, too. Another fear is changes in lipids and cardiovascular risks associated with testosterone. Can you expand on that a little?

MS: The available data indicate that testosterone replacement therapy within the physiologic range by transdermal or injectable testosterone preparation is not associated with worsening of the lipid profile. Studies using physiologic replacement doses of testosterone show no change, or only a slight decrease, in HDL, often with a reduction in total cholesterol. The oral non-aromatizable anabolic steroids appear to lower high-density lipoprotein (HDL) levels.

The belief that testosterone is a risk factor for cardiac disease is based on the observation that men have both a higher incidence of cardiovascular events and higher testosterone levels than women do. There is little data for this idea. Many studies suggest the opposite. There are multiple studies showing a relation between hypogonadism and an increased cardiovascular risk.

There is evidence that testosterone replacement therapy may be beneficial for men with cardiac disease. In a small study, men with chronic stable angina who were treated with transdermal testosterone replacement therapy had greater angina free exercise tolerance. Importantly, testosterone replacement therapy has not shown an increased incidence of cardiovascular disease or stroke.

NV: There are some data on hypogonadism and increased risks of cardiovascular events. Is that what you mean? Some people actually become so severely hypogonadal, they actually may be risking higher incidence of heart attacks and strokes?

MS: That is correct. There are numerous studies demonstrating the relationship between low testosterone levels and adverse cardiovascular events, as well as stroke. Also, there are case study reports of people who stop anabolic steroids, and then suffer a heart attack.

In the book that I wrote, one of the studies in the published literature, looking at the effects of anabolic steroids in certain populations, for 12 weeks, did not look at the patients after they stopped the drug. If you want to look at the effects of these drugs, you need to see what happens when you stop them. I filed a Freedom of Information Act to obtain the patient records. One of the patients actually suffered a heart attack within four weeks of stopping the anabolic steroid. The details, including the original patient records, of this case are reported in my book.

NV: Should patients with an increased or elevated prostatic specific antigen (PSA) avoid testosterone? What role does testosterone replacement therapy (TRT) have on prostate cancer, if any? Is there a risk of worsening prostate cancer with TRT?

MS: You brought up a number of important and controversial issues. It is generally agreed that TRT with established prostate cancer is contraindicated.

It is known that suppression of testosterone levels causes regression of prostate cancer, and it is now commonplace for men with metastatic prostate cancer to undergo treatment designed to lower testosterone levels. The question becomes if lowering testosterone causes prostate cancer to regress, does elevating testosterone cause prostate cancer to appear?

There are case reports suggesting that TRT may convert an occult cancer into a clinically apparent lesion. These studies are wrong. One must be very careful in attributing causality to testosterone, since over 200,000 men are given a diagnosis of prostate cancer each year, and most of these cases are first detected by a rise in the PSA level unrelated to testosterone therapy. Studies have demonstrated a low frequency of prostate cancer in association with TRT. Despite extensive research, there is no compelling evidence that testosterone has a causative role in prostate cancer.

There appears to be no compelling evidence at present to suggest that men with higher testosterone levels are at greater risk of prostate cancer or treating men who have hypogonadism with exogenous androgens increases this risk. In fact, prostate cancer becomes more prevalent exactly at the time of a man's life when testosterone levels decline.

Little evidence exists on the safety of TRT initiation after treatment for primary prostate cancer. In one very small case series, TRT after treatment of organ confined prostate cancer produced no adverse effects. There are no large, long-term studies proving that the risk of recurrence is not affected by TRT. Personally, I would be reluctant to provide TRT in prostate cancer; treatment should be left to strict research protocols.

PSA is a serum glycoprotein made by the normal prostate that is widely used as a tumor marker, because elevated PSA levels correlate with the risk of prostate cancer. A PSA value greater than 4.0 ng/mL has been the standard indication for prostate biopsy since the introduction of this test in the 1980s.

Testosterone trials have inconsistently shown a rise in PSA, typically between 0.2 and 0.5 ng/mL. A greater increase in PSA arouses concern that prostate cancer has developed. It is my practice to recommend a prostate biopsy in any patient with a yearly PSA increase of 1.0 ng/mL or more. If the PSA level increases by 0.75 ng/mL in one year, I repeat the PSA measurement in three to six months and recommend a biopsy if there is any further increase.

NV: Can you explain what polycythemia is and what it means when it comes to cardiovascular risk and other issues?

MS: In respect to anabolic steroid-induced polycythemia, polycythemia is a condition that results in an increased level of circulating red blood cells in the blood stream. Erythrocytosis is a more specific term that is used to denote increased red blood cells. People with polycythemia have an increase in hematocrit, hemoglobin, or red blood cell count above the normal limits. The reporting of polycythemia is typically in terms of increased hematocrit or hemoglobin.

Hematocrit is a blood test that measures the percentage of red blood cells found in the whole blood. This measurement depends on the number and size of red blood cells. Normally, for a male, the hematocrit raises up to a level of 52–54 depending on the reporting laboratory reference range. Polycythemia is considered when the hematocrit is greater than the upper limit of normal.

Hemoglobin is the protein molecule in red blood cells that carries oxygen from the lungs to the body's tissues and returns carbon dioxide from the tissues to the lungs. The hemoglobin level is expressed as the amount of hemoglobin in grams (g) per deciliter (dl) of the whole blood, a deciliter being 100 mL, for adult males: 14–18 gm/dL. Polycythemia is considered when a hemoglobin level is greater than 18 g/dL in men.

It is a thickening of the blood. The blood becomes almost like sludge. You would think that with the increased number of red blood cells, it would carry more oxygen; but its oxygen-carrying capacity decreases markedly. Without treatment, polycythemia can be life threatening. Elevation above the normal range may have grave consequences, particularly in the elderly, since an attendant increase in blood viscosity could aggravate vascular disease in the coronary, cerebrovascular, or peripheral vascular circulation. However, with proper medical care, many people experience few problems related to this disease.

Symptoms of polycythemia can be none to minimal in many people.

Some general and nonspecific symptoms include weakness, fatigue, headache, itching, redness of your skin, bruising, joint pain, dizziness, abdominal pain, shortness of breath, breathing difficulty when you lie down; and numbness, tingling, or burning in the hands, feet, arms, or legs.

NV: Or when they work out, they turn red.

MS: That can certainly be a symptom of polycythemia.

NV: Is the incidence of polycythemia related to the route of administration, dose, duration, and age? Is polycythemia common in replacement doses?

MS: Yes. It occurs quite frequently in people who are just on replacement testosterone. Older men appear more sensitive to the erythropoietic effects of testosterone than young men do. Both testosterone dose and mode of delivery affect the magnitude of hematocrit elevation.

The incidence of testosterone-associated polycythemia may be lower in males receiving pharmacokinetically steady-state delivery of testosterone formulations, than it is in receiving intramuscular injections.

In patients using topical preparations, there is a 5–20 percent incidence of erythrocytosis. There is an apparent direct relation between testosterone dosage and the incidence of erythrocytosis. Erythrocytosis occurs in about 5–15 percent by patches and in 10–20 percent with gel preparations depending on the use of 50 mg/day (delivering 5 mg /day) and 100 mg/day (delivering 10 mg/day) during the course of approximately 14 year.

The most commonly used forms of intramuscular-injectable testosterone esters are testosterone enanthate and cypionate. Injectable testosterone esters generate supranormal testosterone levels shortly after injection and then testosterone levels decline very rapidly, becoming subnormal in the days before the next injection.

Testosterone ester injections have been reported to be associated with a higher risk of erythrocytosis than transdermal testosterone. It is unclear whether the higher frequency of erythrocytosis observed with injectable testosterone esters is due to the higher dose of testosterone delivered by the injections or the higher peaks of testosterone levels. In one study, intramuscular injections of testosterone enanthate produced an elevated hematocrit over 40 percent.

NV: Is therapeutic phlebotomy a good way to manage polycythemia?

MS: Untoward events are unlikely with mild erythrocytosis of relatively short duration. Therapeutic phlebotomy and blood donation are overall a safe procedure, the frequency of side effects being low and their severity weak. Other options include dosage reduction or the withholding of testosterone. However, these latter options can be problematic since the patient will experience symptoms of anabolic steroid-induced hypogonadism.

This does present a catch-22 for many physicians. Because the half-life of the red blood cell is approximately 120 days, it might be a considerable length of time, more than three months or longer, to normalize the hemoglobin or hematocrit upon TRT cessation. But, the problem of anabolic steroid-induced hypogonadism symptoms complicated matters.

Many a times, an attempt will be to maintain TRT while simultaneously performing a therapeutic phlebotomy. Because of the increased erythropoiesis, production of red blood cells, it feels like the proverbial chasing one's tail. In a number of therapeutic phlebotomies, the units of the blood that have to be taken off are clearly quite excessive; and we do not want to do that too quickly. It may come to be three, four, or even five pints of blood that have to be taken off.

In order to get a good hold on the problem of polycythemia, it will be necessary to discontinue TRT. What we have done again, in our protocol, is that we have stopped the testosterone, thereby removing the cause of the increased red blood cell production, treat them with the HPTA protocol that prevents the hypogonadism, and have the therapeutic phlebotomy done. They are able to get the hemoglobin or hematocrit down to the normal level, do not go through the adverse effects of the hypogonadism; and then, at the other end, be able to start the testosterone therapy again. As far as we can determine, no testosterone associated thromboembolic events have been reported to date.

NV: I am actually surprised how many patients are out there that do not have their physician following up their hematocrit when they are put on testosterone or anabolics for wasting syndrome. It is something that the physician should be looking out for and measuring.

MS: The hemoglobin and hematocrit is part of the routine laboratory follow-up for anyone on TRT. If a patient complains of any of the symptoms we describe for polycythemia, a hemoglobin and hematocrit should be checked. One of the confounding problems is the symptoms tend to be nonspecific.

NV: Can you say something about the prophylactic use of finasteride or dutasteride to avoid DHT-related problems like prostate enlargement or hair loss? Is there a role for the use of finasteride or dutasteride to prevent the possible increase of hair loss with TRT?

MS: Finasteride and dutasteride are 5-alpha reductase inhibitors. 5-alpha reductase comes in two forms, type 1 and type 2, and is responsible for the conversion of testosterone into DHT. Finasteride inhibits type 2 only while dutasteride inhibits both forms.

Finasteride comes in two doses depending on whether the indication is for hair loss or benign prostate hypertrophy. Propecia, 1 mg, is for hair loss. Proscar, 5 mg, is for prostatic hypertrophy.

DHT has been shown to be important in the development of hair loss or male pattern baldness. I am unaware any studies indicating a worsening of hair loss or male pattern baldness, though this possibility has not been carefully studied. There are anecdotal reports. The prophylactic use of these drugs is an individual decision after weighing the risks and benefits.

DHT is also important in prostate health. It is thought an overabundance of DHT may be important in benign prostatic hyperplasia (BPH) and prostate cancer. Dutasteride provides greater suppression of DHT than finasteride does, thereby underlying the hypothesis that inhibition of both type 1 and type 2 would provide correspondingly greater protection than inhibition of type 2 alone.

However, significant side effects of finasteride use include reduced volume of ejaculate, erectile dysfunction, loss of libido, and gynecomastia. This will prevent many from their use.

Some people think that DHT will affect lean body composition. DHT does have a higher affinity for the androgen receptor. But the enzyme that converts testosterone into DHT is not located in the muscle. There is no evidence for these drugs to effect muscle mass.

NV: What about other issues related TRT, such as to increased estrogen levels and gynecomastia?

MS: A small number report breast tenderness and swelling. Fluid retention is uncommon and generally mild, but TRT should be used cautiously in men with congestive heart failure or renal insufficiency. After confirmation of elevated estrogen, estradiol, levels, this can be treated with either an aromatization inhibitor or estradiol receptor blocker. This must be done very carefully as any prolonged reduction in estradiol levels runs the risk of causing osteoporosis.

Exacerbation of sleep apnea or the development of sleep apnea has been associated with TRT who have other identifiable risk factors for sleep apnea. The mechanism appears to be central mediated rather than by means of changes in the airway. Other side effects include acne, oily skin, increased body hair, and flushing. Hypertension has rarely been reported.

Of course, the adverse effect I am most concerned with is androgen-induced hypogonadism, which occurs in one hundred percent of individuals stopping TRT, the variables being the duration and severity.

On testosterone replacement therapy, for those without organic hypogonadism, those with late onset of hypogonadism, the only thing that I always caution about is that people should not be on testosterone replacement therapy, year after year after year, without stopping every 12–18 months to restore the axis, to make sure the function is still there. The longer you are on testosterone, the harder it is going to be to come off testosterone.

NV: In your opinion, can you tell us a little bit about the different options for TRT? Have you seen any difference in using gels versus injections? Is there any advantage or disadvantage to using either one?

MS: Injectable, transdermal, buccal, and oral testosterone formulations are available for clinical use. These forms of treatment differ in several key areas.

Oral preparations include methyl testosterone and fluoxymesterone, which are rarely prescribed because of their association with substantial liver toxicity. In Europe, there is an oral preparation of testosterone undecanoate, Andriol. It has a poor history of bioavailability.

Recently, the FDA approved a buccal preparation of testosterone, Striant. Striant requires administration twice a day. It is used little at this time.

Transdermal testosterone is available as a patch, Testim, and gel, Androgel. Daily application is required for each of these. They are designed to deliver 5–10 mg of testosterone a day. The advantages include ease of use and maintenance of relatively uniform serum testosterone levels over time. Skin irritation in the form of itching and redness is a frequent adverse effect of Testim with reports as high as 60–70 percent. This is uncommon with Androgel. Inadequate absorption through the skin may limit the value of transdermal preparations in some persons. A common problem is the low dose preparations provide inadequate serum testosterone levels. This is also seen with the high dose.

The topical have become, by far, the most-used products in the last decade or so, approaching a billion dollars in sales. Androgel is the biggest product of the topical.

If the patient is not too scared of doing injectables, oil-based testosterone ester preparations are available. The most commonly used injectables are Delatestryl or testosterone enanthate and depo testosterone or testosterone cypionate. In my practice, the typical dose is between 100 and 150 mg/week. The peak serum levels occur in 2–5 days after injection, and a return to baseline is usually observed 10 days after injection. In this manner, adequate serum levels are maintained. Intramuscular injections of testosterone can cause local pain, soreness, bruising, redness, swelling, and possible infection.

NV: Most doctors prescribe 1-cc of 200 mL of testosterone every two weeks. Can you describe the problems with this schedule, if any?

MS: This is a problem that is seen much more often than necessary. Many doctors use a typical dose is 100 mg/week or 200–300 mg every two to three weeks.

Within 7–10 days after injection, the serum testosterone levels are low to abnormally low. This is described as a "roller coaster" effect, characterized by alternating periods of symptomatic benefit and a return to baseline symptoms, corresponding to the fluctuations in serum testosterone levels. This can be discovered by having the testosterone level checked within 24 hours prior to injection.

NV: Can you talk to us a little bit about compounding pharmacy products? In particular, when using testosterone gels with concentrations higher than 1 percent for reaching total testosterone blood levels above 500 ng/L. Have you had any experience with the compounding industry?

MS: I have had some experience with the compounding industry.

Compounding pharmacies are very capable at providing higher concentrations of transdermal testosterone preparations. Because of this, they are able to supply a transdermal product in small volumes. They also tend to be less expensive than commercially available pharmaceutical testosterone replacement options.

NV: Do you think it is advisable to get your testosterone levels rechecked after a few weeks of starting any of the therapies?

MS: My protocol is that once I start a patient on testosterone, I check the testosterone level 4–6 weeks after initiating TRT. In patients using topical preparations, I recommend testing within 4–6 hours after application. Those using injectables of testosterone esters, I recommend testing within 24 hours before their next scheduled injection.

NV: Do you have any preference between the free testosterone and total testosterone test?

MS: In the monitoring of the patient on TRT, I utilize the total testosterone. The initial evaluation of a patient might include the use of free testosterone or bioavailable testosterone. In a symptomatic individual, the total testosterone can be normal but the free or bioavailable testosterone abnormal.

Testosterone circulates in three forms. Testosterone circulates in a free or unbound state, tightly bound to SHBG, or weakly bound to the blood protein albumin. Bioavailable, non-SHBG, testosterone includes free testosterone and testosterone that is bound to albumin but does not include SHBG -bound testosterone.

Examined changes over time have demonstrated a decrease in the total testosterone and an increase in SHBG levels. Because of this, the total testosterone might be normal, whereas the free or bioavailable testosterone is abnormal. If these alternative methods are used to diagnose hypogonadism, their utility during TRT is limited.

I would caution about the assay methodology used to calculate the free or bioavailable testosterone. The methods used to conduct the measurements vary in their accuracy, standardization, the extent of validation, and the reproducibility of results.

Bioavailable testosterone is measured or calculated in several ways. SHBG bound testosterone can be precipitated with ammonium sulfate and the remaining testosterone is then taken as the bioavailable.

Measures of free testosterone (FT) are controversial. The only standardized and validated method is equilibrium dialysis or by calculating free testosterone levels based on separate measurements of testosterone and SHBG. Other measures of free testosterone are less accurate.

NV: And your goal is usually to have patients above what level?

MS: I like their total testosterone trough or lower level to be in the 500–700 range, normal being 300–1,000 ng/dL.

NV: Besides checking of the initial T level, can you elaborate on the monitoring during TRT?

MS: I recommend a periodic follow-up of patients receiving replacement testosterone therapy at the interval of three months during the first year of treatment. Afterward, patients are followed up every six months. It is important to do a review of systems to ensure the relief of the complaining symptoms as well as no worsening or new symptoms.

In addition to the serum total testosterone, I routinely monitor the basic chemistry profile, which includes liver function, kidney function, electrolytes, glucose, lipid panel, and hemoglobin or hematocrit. At three months, I will often include estradiol and DHT levels.

If the patient is older than 50 years, I include the PSA. The role of digital rectal examination (DRE) and PSA in detecting early, clinically significant, prostate cancer is controversial. I discuss this with each patient and allow them to decide on their use.

NV: How about the new non-steroidal androgens that are in the pipeline? Can you tell us what you have read about them?

MS: They are called SARM: selective androgen receptor modulators. They are going to become more and more popular. The closest SARM that is coming to the market, and it is years away, is called ostarine. It is being developed by GTx, Inc. Ligand Pharmaceuticals has a SARM in early phase of development. They are both traded on the NASDAQ Exchange.

The initial studies are being done in cancer patients. The data collected is change in muscle mass and strength. The clinical outcome being measured is the six-minute walk test.

My feeling on this is that we have a long way to go before these things come to market. If they come to market within the next 5–10 years, we will be lucky. As far as I know, these are the only SARMs in human clinical trials.

NV: I have also heard that SARMs may not have any influence on sexual function, only on lean body mass and maybe some functional capacity. They are really not replacement of testosterone. Are they?

MS: From the initial studies, these are meant to take the place of anabolic steroids, not testosterone. There are no indications SARMs are being developed as TRT. The data from both animal and human studies is that they act similarly, if not identically, to anabolic steroids. They act through the androgen receptor. They do cause HPTA suppression.

Even though they have the same effect, they will be able to be marketed without that name "anabolic steroids." This would be an obvious advantage in their marketing. It should be noted that these drugs, SARMs, have already found their way into the nonprescription or illicit market.

NV: Can somebody on testosterone replacement become less fertile? If a man wants to impregnate his wife after, let us say, a year of testosterone replacement, is there any risk for that man to become less fertile to his wife?

MS: Testicular size and consistency often diminish, and men should be advised that fertility would be greatly compromised during testosterone replacement therapy because of downregulation of LH and FSH.

The general rule is they will become less fertile. But you cannot depend on its use as a fertility drug. And that is where we come in with contraceptive studies. We have many, many contraceptive studies that use testosterone cypionate at 200 mg a week and find that, yes, it decreases fertility. But there is still a subset of men that still produce sperm that are fertile.

NV: Are these men good candidates for a protocol to reset their HPGA?
MS: We have had many men who come to the clinic with the actual complaint that they were using anabolic steroids, or they were using testosterone, and they now want to get their wife pregnant. Although many will return to normal after stopping TRT, this period can be

lengthy.

The amazing thing to me is that the number of people that come to me, who have seen the doctor, who are either non-prescription or prescription anabolic steroid users, testosterone with or without combination of anabolic steroids, who have the problem of infertility; and their doctors have no idea what to do, except to do nothing. But on top of this are all the psychological problems and effects that come along with doing nothing as a consequence of anabolic steroid-induced hypogonadism. The HPTA protocol has restored fertility as well as decreased the time substantially.

NV: Can you expand about resetting the HPGA?

MS: The word resetting is a misnomer, though recent studies published in the *New England Journal of Medicine* (NEJM) do indicate this possible. In 2007, the *NEJM* reports on the resetting of the HPTA after TRT for adult onset idiopathic hypogonadism. This is the first report demonstrating HPTA plasticity in adulthood. The term I prefer is HPTA functionality and restoration.

There are clear conditions under which testosterone requires administration for life-long treatment. However, there are increasing numbers of individuals being treated with TRT who do not fall under these disorders. TRT is being prescribed more and more for late onset hypogonadism. This is called by many other names, including andropause, androgen deficiency of the aging male, and others.

There are no consequences of the decline in serum testosterone with age that are known with certainty. Several parallels exist between the effects of aging and those of hypogonadism, which suggest that the decline in serum testosterone might be a cause of several effects of aging. Since the long-term effects of androgen treatment for late onset hypogonadism or andropause are not well-known, I discontinue therapy on an approximate annual basis to ensure HPTA normalization—functionality. This allows the patient the autonomy to stop therapy should the need arise.

What is clear is that upon stopping testosterone or anabolic steroids, a period of anabolic steroid-induced hypogonadism ensues. This occurs in one hundred percent of individuals stopping testosterone. The only variables are the duration and severity. The duration of hypogonadism, or the severity of hypogonadism, is typically related to the anabolic steroid drug, dose, and duration.

In other words, one person that is on testosterone for an entire year;

they may come back to normal within 1 or 2 months. Another person may take 12, 18 months, or even 3 years to come back to normal. The best studies we have on this are contraceptive studies with testosterone for over a year. And what we find in those studies is that it may take up to three years for a person to return to normal.

If they have been taking those anabolic steroids to improve their body composition, increase the lean body mass, and decrease the body fat, that all goes back to normal after stopping anabolic steroids. But you are also going to be exposed to the other adverse effects of hypogonadism, which include adverse psychological and cardiovascular effects. Some of the adverse psychological effects are depression, decreased cognitive abilities, insomnia, decreased libido, and erection dysfunction. More significantly, after cessation adds the comorbid condition of hypogonadism to their already existing chronic illness.

AAS, including testosterone, licit and illicit, administration induces a state of hypogonadism that continues after their cessation. All compounds classified as androgens or anabolic steroids cause a negative feedback inhibition of the hypothalamic-pituitary testicular axis, suppress endogenous gonadotropin secretion, and as a consequence serum testosterone.

The symptoms of AIH are identical to classical hypogonadism. This problem prevents many of discontinuing testosterone or anabolic steroids. As we have said, there are many reasons for stopping testosterone, including polycythemia, gynecomastia, and other issue as compliance, affordability, and changing life style.

The accepted standard of care within the medical community for anabolic steroid induced hypogonadism is to do nothing with the expectation the individual will return to normal unassisted. But the literature shows this not to be the case.

AIH is critical toward any planned use of AAS or similar compound to effect positive changes in muscle mass and muscle strength as well as an understanding for what has been termed anabolic steroid dependency. The further understanding and treatments that mitigate or prevent AIH could contribute to androgen therapies for wasting associated diseases and stopping nonprescription AAS use.

NV: What is used for restoring the hormonal axis?
MS: A combination of three drugs. The individual use of HCG, clomiphene citrate, and tamoxifen is well-known, well-accepted, and well-tested standards of care treatments in peer-reviewed

medical literature for diagnostic testing for underlying pathology of hypogonadism. The HPTA protocol uses the medications human chorionic gonadotropin, clomiphene citrate, and tamoxifen.

The first phase of the HPTA protocol examines the functionality of the testicles by the direct action of HCG. HCG raises sex hormone levels directly through the stimulation of the testes and secondly decreases the production and level of gonadotropin LH. The increase in serum testosterone with the HCG stimulation is useful in determining whether any primary testicular dysfunction is present.

This initial value is a measure of the ability of the testicles to respond to stimulation from HCG. Demonstration of the HPTA functionality is an adequate response of the testicles to raise the serum level of T well into the normal range. If this is observed, HCG is discontinued. The failure of the testes to respond to an HCG challenge is indicative of primary testicular failure. In the simplest terms, the first half of the protocol is to determine testicular production and reserve by direct stimulation with HCG. If one is unable to obtain adequate (normal) levels successfully in the first half, there is little cause or reason to proceed to the second half.

The second phase of the HPTA protocol, clomiphene and tamoxifen, examines the ability of the hypothalamic-pituitary axis to respond to stimulation by producing LH levels within the normal reference range. The clomiphene citrate challenge differentiates secondary hypogonadism. Clomiphene is an antiestrogen, which decreases the estrogen effect in the body. It has a dual effect by stimulating the hypothalamic pituitary area and it has an antiestrogenic effect, so that it decreases the effect of estrogen in the body. Tamoxifen is more of a strict antiestrogen; it decreases the effect of estrogen in the body, and potentiates the action of clomiphene. Tamoxifen and clomiphene citrate compete with estrogen for estrogen receptor binding sites, thus eliminating excess estrogen circulation at the level of the hypothalamus and pituitary, allowing gonadotropin production to resume. Administering them together produces an elevation of LH and secondarily gonadal sex hormones. The administration of clomiphene leads to an appropriate rise in the levels of LH, suggesting that the negative feedback control on the hypothalamus is intact and that the storage and release of gonadotropins by the pituitary is normal. If there was a successful stimulation of testicular T levels by HCG, but an inadequate or no response in LH production, then the patient has hypogonadotropic, secondary, hypogonadism.

In the simplest terms, the second half of the protocol is to determine hypothalamo-pituitary production and reserve with clomiphene and tamoxifen. The physiological type of hypogonadism—hypogonadotropic or secondary—is characterized by abnormal low or low normal gonadotropin (LH) production in response to clomiphene citrate and tamoxifen. In the functional type of hypogonadism, the ability to stimulate the HPTA to produce LH and T levels within the normal reference range occurs.

There is a dearth of good studies in anabolic steroids, both while you are taking them and after you stop them, I think this is going to be something that we are going to need to look at in the future. In fact, we are going to plan on looking at it in our proposed clinical studies that we have with our company for the prevention of anabolic steroid-induced hypogonadism.

Dr. Michael Scally can be contacted at mscally@alum.mit.edu. His book "Anabolic Steroids - A Question of Muscle: Human Subject Abuses in Anabolic Steroid Research" is available on Amazon.com

-APPENDIX A-
Confidential Medical History Form
(Courtesy of Dr. John Crisler- allthingsmale.com)

WE REALIZE THIS MEDICAL HISTORY FORM IS SOMEWHAT LONG. HOWEVER, IT IS ABSOLUTELY NECESSARY FOR US TO EVALUATE YOUR GENERAL HEALTH AND SAFELY AND LEGITIMATELY PRESCRIBE THE MEDICATIONS YOU WANT AND NEED. MAKE SURE TO TAKE A FEW MINUTES TO CAREFULLY AND COMPLETELY ANSWER <u>EVERY</u> QUESTION. FAILING TO DO SO WILL PREVENT US FROM HELPING YOU, AS DOING SO COULD POSSIBLY JEOPARDIZE YOUR HEALTH. DO THE BEST YOU CAN-WE WILL FOLLOW-UP WITH ANY QUESTIONS WE MAY HAVE. REMEMBER, THIS INFORMATION IS COMPLETELY CONFIDENTIAL.

Please initial here that you have read the above statement:

I am a NEW /ESTABLISHED patient (circle one).

1. First name:
2. Middle name:
3. Last name:
4. Address:
5. City:
6. State:
7. Zip code:
8. Shipping address (if different than address above):
9. City:
10. State:
11. Zip code:

CONTACT INFORMATION

12. Email:
13. Repeat Email Address [to confirm]:
14. Daytime phone:
15. Night time phone:

PERSONAL INFORMATION

16.   Birth date:
17.   Driver's License Number:
18.   Social Security Number:
19.   Marital Status (Married, Divorced, Never Married, Gay)
20.   Sex:
21.   Height:
22.   Weight:
23.   Occupation:
24.   Medical Insurance Provider and member ID:
25.   Prescription Insurance Provider and member ID:
26.   Do you have a primary care physician?
27.   When was your last complete physical examination?
28.   What were the results of that exam?
29.   Will you have a copy of that report and any labs sent to us (mail or FAX)?
30.   (FOR OVER 40) Did you have your prostate examined?
31.   (FOR OVER 40) Did you have your PSA checked? If so, what was it?

PAST MEDICAL HISTORY

Please indicate if you now have, or have EVER had:

32.   Anemia
33.   Arthritis
34.   Asthma
35.   Blood disease
36.   Bronchitis
37.   Diabetes
38.   Emphysema
39.   Epilepsy
40.   Gout
41.   Hepatitis
42.   Heart disease
43.   High blood pressure
44.   High cholesterol
45.   Kidney disease
46.   Migraines
47.   Mononucleosis
48.   Pneumonia
49.   Psychological problems
50.   Rheumatic fever
51.   Seizures

52.　　Stroke
53.　　Thyroid disease
54.　　TB
55.　　Ulcers
56.　　Urinary tract infections
57.　　Have you ever had any form of cancer?
　　　　　　If so, please detail:

PAST SURGICAL HISTORY
What surgeries have you had?

58.　　Appendectomy
59.　　Cholecystectomy (gall bladder removal)
60.　　Mastectomy (removal of breast material-usually for
　　　　gynecomastia)
61.　　Tonsillectomy
62.　　Prostatectomy
63.　　Hernia repair
64.　　Other surgeries (please explain):

65.　　Have you ever been hospitalized (other than for the above
　　　　mentioned surgeries)? If so, please list the reason and give
　　　　approximate　　date(s):

FAMILY MEDICAL HISTORY
Have your brothers and/or sisters, parents or grandparents, ever had
(Please tell which family member(s)?

66.　　Heart attack
67.　　Diabetes
68.　　Kidney disease
69.　　Leukemia
70.　　Mental disorders
71.　　Stroke
72.　　Prostate cancer
73.　　Other cancer

Please detail ANY of the above:

74.　　Are you allergic to anything?
75.　　If yes, what?
76.　　Do you smoke?
77.　　If so, how much each day?
78.　　How long have you smoked?

79.   Do you drink alcohol?
       How many drinks do you typically have in a week?
80.   Do you use any illicit substances (get high)?
       If so, which ones?

REVIEW OF SYSTEMS
<u>Do you CURRENTLY have (please circle)?</u>:

81.   Head aches
82.   Vision changes
83.   Hearing changes
84.   Chronic sinusitis
85.   Allergic sinus problems
86.   Any tenderness or sores in your mouth or throat
87.   Bloody noses
88.   Chronic cough
89.   Do you spit up blood?
90.   Shortness of breath
91.   Chest pain
92.   Dizziness
93.   Congestive heart failure
94.   Palpitations
95.   Any form of arrythmia
96.   Heart murmur
97.   Recurring constipation
98.   Recurring diarrhea
99.   Gallbladder disease
100.   Throw up blood
101.   Blood in your stool or black tarry stool
102.   Hernia
103.   Loss of appetite
104.   Indigestion
105.   Nausea
106.   Vomiting
107.   Jaundice (yellow skin)
108.   Do your eyes look yellow?
109.   Do you have abdominal pain?
       If so, please describe and tell where:
110.   Pancreatitis
111.   Do you urinate alright?
112.   Does it hurt when you urinate?
113.   Is there any blood in your urine?
114.   Have you ever had a STD (Sexually Transmitted Disease)?
115.   Tingling in your fingers or toes

116. Acne
     Describe any acne history:
117. Do you ever pass out?
118. Do you have cold intolerance?
119. Do you bruise easily?
120. Depression
121. Anxiety
122. Decreased sexual potency
     If so, is this causing stress in your relationship?
123. Sleep disturbances
124. Generalized muscle aches and pains
125. Joint pain
126. Back pain
127. Fatigue
128. Lethargy
129. Nocturnal emissions
130. Sensitive or swollen nipples?
131. Did you have swollen or painful nipples BEFORE you ever used steroids (for Steroid Consult only)?
131. Can you feel any lumps around your nipples
132. Are you losing your hair? Were you losing it before you started using steroids (AAS Consult only)? If so, is it falling out more quickly now?

GENERAL
134. Loss of appetite
135. Unexplained weight loss
136. Do you consider yourself to be in good health?
137. Do you sleep well?
     Average hours of sleep per night:
138. Do you regularly self examine your testicles?
139. Tell me about your diet (Details please)

MEDICATIONS

140. Do you take any prescription medications (other than steroids)?
     If so, please list, and give dosages:
141. What supplements do you take (vitamins, minerals, neutraceuticals, etc.)? List all (with amounts or dosages) each day.
142. How much water do you usually drink each day?

QUESTIONS FOR STEROID CONSULT ONLY (for confidential information only- We do not prescribe these agents for non medical uses)

143.   Tell us, as accurately as you can which steroids you are going to take, or have taken, for THIS cycle (AAS Consult only):
144.   How many times have you been on a steroid cycle (if any)?
145.   How long ago was your first steroid cycle (if any)?
146.   How long was your break before starting this cycle?
147.   Describe your past usage, if any, of hCG, Nolvadex, Clomid, Arimidex or finasteride:
148.   Have you ever had any problems (side effects) with any of the medications mentioned in question #147 If so, please describe:
149.   Which of the ancillaries are you looking for, and how much of each do you want (AAS Consult only)? This question is for experienced AAS users only.

HRT patients only (questions 150-159):

150.   Do you plan on having more children?
151.   Do you have a decrease in sex drive?
152.   If the answer to #151 is "YES", is this affecting your relationship?
153.   Has your strength or endurance decreased?
154.   Are you enjoying life less?
155.   Are you sad or grumpy?
156.   Are your erections less strong?
157.   Has your work performance decreased?
158.   Do you have a hard time recovering from physical activity?
159.   Have you ever been on HRT before?

CONGRATULATIONS! YOU ARE (FINALLY!) DONE WITH THIS FORM

I HAVE COMPLETED THE MEDICAL HISTORY FORM TO THE BEST OF MY KNOWLEDGE. I CERTIFY THAT MY ANSWERS ARE COMPLETE, HONEST AND

Signed: _____

Date: ....

-APPENDIX B-

Resources and Patient Assistance Programs

Internet Discussion Groups

Subscribe to a yahoo group that discusses testosterone replacement by sending an email to MensHealthAdvances-subscribe@yahoogroups.com

Another good web site to join is: www.mesomorphosis.com. There you can join forums on testosterone, exercise, nutrition, supplements, and other topics related to fitness.

On Facebook, I have created a page called "Testosterone Replacement Discussion group". Please search those key words and join us!

I will be posting updates on **TestosteroneWisdom.com** frequently on latest developments in the field and also my own experiences.

Patient Assistance Programs

Testim
If you have insurance but it charges you a high copayment for the drug, you can apply for co-pay assistance. If you have questions about this program please contact the Testim Voucher Hotline at 1-877-217-5737.

Testim's copy program is not valid for claims submitted by or on behalf of a patient for reimbursement or coverage for Testim under Medicaid, Medicare, or other federal or state government health care programs. Not valid in conjunction with any 3rd party payer program in Massachusetts. https://www.trialcard.com/WebRebate/Testim2008/

For men who do not have insurance and meet the financial criteria, the following information can guide them on how to apply for free product.

Program Name	Auxilium Patient Assistance Program
Program Address	40 Valley Stream Parkway Malvem, PA 19355
Phone Number	877-663-0412
Fax Number	866-837-7293
Medications on Program	Testim 1% Gel 1% gel 50 mg (testosterone topical)
Application Forms	Auxilium Patient Assistance Program: www.needymeds.org/papforms/auxili0462.pdf
Online Application	No on-line application available at this time
Eligibility Guidelines and Notes	The patient must have no prescription coverage for the requested medication and have an income at or below $23,660 per individual, $29,140 for 2 people, $36,620 for 3 people, $44,100 for 4 people, etc. The patient must have a diagnosis of hypogonadism. The patient must also reside in the US. Patients must be male. Patients who were eligible for Medicare Part D, but did not enroll may still be eligible for this program. Patients who enrolled in Medicare Part D, but are in the Donut Hole are not eligible. Applicants that do not qualify under the program's set criteria may still apply by completing the "Hardship Exception Request" section of the application form.

Application Process	Anyone requesting assistance can call to request a faxed application or download it from the website. The application will be faxed out. The completed application must be mailed back. The patient is notified of eligibility for the program. The decision is made at meetings that occur approximately every month. (Speak to the company for specifics.) The medication is shipped within 4-6 weeks of receiving the application.
Application Requirements	The doctor must fill out a section, sign the application and attach a prescription for 6 months. The patient must fill out a section, sign the application and attach a denial letter from Medicaid.
Program Details	A six-month supply is sent to the doctor's office. The company automatically sends out refills. Every six months a new application is needed with a new prescription, once a year an application with documentation is needed.

Androgel

If you have insurance but your co-pay is too high, you can apply for a co-pay assistance by visiting:
https://webrebate.trialcard.com/coupon/androgelportal/QuizPrescribe.aspx

If you do not have insurance and meet the financial criteria, you can get the product for free. Here is the information to apply:

Program Name	Solvay Pharmaceuticals Patient Assistance Program
Program Address	C/O Express Scripts Specialty Distribution Svc. PO Box 66550 St. Louis MO 63166-6550
Phone Number	800-256-8918
Fax Number	800-276-9901
Medications on Program	Androgel 1% Gel 2.5gm, 5gm (testosterone topical) Androgel 1% Pump (testosterone topical)
Application Forms	Abbott Labs Patient Assistance Program
Online Application	No online application available at this time Form: abbottgrowth-us.com/static/wma/pdf/1/6/1/1/3/SolvayApplication0210.pdf
Eligibility Guidelines and Notes	The patient must have no prescription coverage for any medications and meet income guidelines that are not disclosed. Medical diagnosis necessary for this program is not specified. The patient must also be a US resident. If a patient did not enroll in Medicare Part D, then he may still be eligible for this program and should apply. If a patient has Part D and has been denied coverage, he may be considered by this program.

Application Process	With the patient's permission, anyone concerned can call for an application. The application can be either faxed or mailed out upon request. The completed application must be faxed or mailed from the doctor's office. The doctor or patient should call to check on status. The estimated timeline for acceptance is 7-10 business days. The medication is shipped within 2 business days.
Application Requirements	The doctor must fill out a section and sign the application. The patient must fill out a section, sign the application and attach proof of income.
Program Details	Up to a 90-day supply is sent to the doctor's office. The patient or doctor must contact the company for refills. Once a year a new application with financial documentation is needed.

Bibliography and Further Reading

Bhasin et al. **"Testosterone Therapy in Adult Men with Androgen Deficiency Syndromes: An Endocrine Society Clinical Practice Guideline"**. The Journal of Clinical Endocrinology & Metabolism Vol. 91, No. 6 1995-2010. These are the American Association of Clinical Endocrinologists Medical Guidelines for Clinical Practice for the Evaluation and Treatment of Hypogonadism (You can read them at link 12 and 13 of www.aace.com/pub/guidelines/)

-APPENDIX C-

Compounding Pharmacies

Frequently Asked Questions about Compounding

(This comes from the International Academy of Compounding Pharmacists (IACP) www.iacprx.org)

What is pharmacy compounding?

In general, pharmacy compounding is the customized preparation of a medicine that is not otherwise commercially available. These medications are prescribed by a physician, veterinarian, or other prescribing practitioner, and compounded by a state-licensed pharmacist. A growing number of people and animals have unique health needs that off-the-shelf, one-size-fits-all prescription medicines cannot meet. For them, customized medications are the only way to better health.

Who are compounding pharmacists?

Pharmacy compounding is a centuries-old, well-regulated and common practice. Pharmacists are some of the most respected and trusted professionals in the United States. In a recent survey, pharmacists ranked second (only behind nurses) as the most trusted professionals in American society. Compounding has evolved into a specialty practice within the pharmacy community today. New applications to meet today's patient needs require additional education, equipment, and processes that not all pharmacies possess.

How are compounding pharmacies and pharmacists regulated? Should there be increased federal oversight?

All pharmacies and pharmacists are licensed and strictly regulated at the state level. Compounding is a core component of pharmacy and has always been regulated by state boards, which are constantly updating their standards and regulations. In addition, standards set by the United States Pharmacopeia (USP) are integrated into the practice of pharmacy compounding. The Pharmacy Compounding Accreditation Board (PCAB) has developed national standards to accredit pharmacies that perform a significant amount of compounding.

Does the FDA have the expertise and federal power to regulate compounding pharmacies? Why shouldn't compounded medications, especially the most commonly used combinations, have to go through FDA's established drug approval process?

The medical profession, including the practice of pharmacy, has always been regulated by the states. State boards of pharmacy are in the best position to inspect pharmacy operations, develop appropriate regulations, and respond to problems or violations. The FDA does have an important role to play in making sure that ingredients used in compounding are safe and are manufactured by the FDA-registered and inspected facilities, but there is no such thing as an "FDA-approved" pharmacy.

The FDA's drug approval process takes years and can cost hundreds of millions of dollars. Requiring this for individually personalized medications that fulfill an individual doctor's prescription is both impractical and contrary to the best interests of patients requiring immediate treatment.

What suppliers sell ingredients to compounding pharmacies? How are these suppliers regulated?

Just like big pharmaceutical manufacturing companies, compounding pharmacies get their ingredients for medications from the suppliers that are registered and inspected by the FDA. Foreign suppliers are FDA-registered facilities.

There are thousands of FDA-approved drugs on the market for just about any ailment. Why do we still need compounded medications?

Some valuable medications and their different delivery methods are only available by compounding. Restricting a doctor's access to compounded medications would be a serious mistake. Moreover, because of the economics of pharmaceutical manufacturing, FDA-approved drugs that serve a limited population are often discontinued by manufacturers. In most of these cases the only option left for doctors and their patients is to have a compounding pharmacist make the discontinued drug from scratch using pharmaceutical grade ingredients.

Are compounded medications safe? How does one know that the compounded medication they are taking is safe and effective?

Compounded medications are similar to the so-called off-label use of FDA-approved drugs. When the FDA approves a specific drug as safe and effective, this determination applies only to the specific disease or condition for which the drug was tested. But physicians and veterinarians often prescribe medications for treatments for which they have not been specifically approved. Medical professionals do this because, in their judgment, the treatment is in the best interest of the individual patient.

Similarly, medical professionals often prescribe compounded medications because they believe it is the best medical option for their patients. It is estimated that one fifth of all prescriptions written for FDA-approved drugs are for uses for which they were not specifically approved.

Some Compounding Pharmacies I Have Used:

This is a very small list of the compounding pharmacies that I have used. There are many more around the country, so I encourage you to Google "compounding pharmacy + your city" to find local ones. The ones listed here ship in the United States and require your physician to call in or fax a prescription. You should call them to compare prices and to provide your credit card and address information. Prices for testosterone products, HCG, TRIMIX, clomiphene (Clomid), anastrazole (Arimidex), and other compounded products can vary widely among compounding pharmacies. If your doctor uses only one compounding pharmacy, tell him or her that you will shop around before committing to theirs as the main source of your products.

For a listing of trusted compounded pharmacies, visit TestosteroneWisdom.com

-APPENDIX D-

Physicians Who Treat Hypogonadism

Most primary care doctors in the United States feel comfortable prescribing testosterone in 2010. After you find a potential doctor, ask some basic questions to determine their level of knowledge about testosterone. Some may feel insulted to be asked questions like these, but if they are it's probably not going to be a good match for you (of course, be nice and diplomatic when asking questions!)-

1. How many men does he/she treat for hypogonadism?
1. Does he/she offer HCG therapy, in addition to testosterone for testicular atrophy? (Many doctors do not know how to use HCG.)
2. Does he/she use Arimidex or tamoxifen to keep estradiol down in case of gynecomastia (enlarged breasts)?
2. Does he/she check for primary or secondary hypogonadism?
3. Does he/she allow patients to self-inject at home?
3. Does he/she work with any compounding pharmacies to access cheaper and customized hormonal products? (As mentioned previously, some doctors worry compounding pharmacies have poor quality control)

Here are several resources that can help you if you need to search for a doctor:

Email me at NelsonVergel@gmail.com to see if I know a doctor in your area.

The Hormone Foundation

The Hormone Foundation, the public education affiliate of The Endocrine Society, is a leading source of hormone-related health information for the public, physicians, allied health professionals and the media. Their mission is to serve as a resource for the public by promoting the prevention, treatment and cure of hormone-related conditions through outreach and education.

The Hormone Foundation's physician referral directory is comprised of over 3,000 members of The Endocrine Society, the largest and most influential organization of endocrinologists in the world. The referral is updated weekly with physicians who are accepting new patients.

To find a specialist near you, please use the search tools below. You can search by ZIP code, state/province, or area of specialty (e.g., diabetes, thyroid, etc.) within the United States and abroad.

www.hormone.org/FindAnEndo/index.cfm

Life Extension Foundation, List of Innovative Doctors:

lef.org/Health-Wellness/InnovativeDoctors/

Women's International Pharmacy- Directory of Doctors:

womensinternational.com/resources_referral.html

College Pharmacy – Directory of Doctors

collegepharmacy.com/community/findaprovider.asp

Medibolics.com, Michael Mooney's HIV-related web site

Doctors in this 3 year old list also treat people who are not HIV positive: www.medibolics.com/physic2.htm

Directory of "anti-aging" worldwide doctors

www.worldhealth.net/pages/directory

-APPENDIX E-

HOW TO JOIN TESTOSTERONE RESEARCH STUDIES

Those of you who want to help advance the understanding of testosterone use for different conditions can join research studies that are currently enrolling. I was amazed to see how many studies are out there! However, none are looking at long term management of side effects like polycythemia with therapeutic phlebotomy, testicular atrophy with long term or cycled HCG therapy, HPGA normalization protocols using HCG+Clomid+estrogen blockers, and other important modalities that are being used by many physicians but with little controlled data.

Remember that some studies have placebo arms. Every study requires for you to read and sign a consent form that should clearly describe the risks and implications in joining the study. Make sure that the private investigator or research nurse overseeing the study explains things to you clearly.

Study to Determine the Long-Term Effects of Testosterone Replacement in Men

Unfortunately, there have been no controlled studies on the long-term use of testosterone replacement in men, even though many of us have been using it for over 20 years.

To answer questions about the long-term effect of testosterone replacement therapy in men the National Institute on Aging, part of the National Institutes of Health, announced in November 2009 the start of a large-scale clinical trial to evaluate the effect of testosterone therapy in older men. Led by researchers at the University of Pennsylvania School of Medicine and conducted at 12 sites across the nation, the testosterone trial involves 800 men aged 65 years and older with low testosterone levels. The testosterone trial includes five separate studies. Men aged 65 years and older with low serum testosterone and at least one hypogonadal condition (anemia, decreased physical function, low vitality, impaired cognition, or reduced sexual function) are randomly assigned to participate in a treatment group or a control group.

Treatment groups are given a testosterone gel that is applied to the torso, abdomen, or upper arms. Control groups will receive a placebo gel. Serum testosterone will be measured monthly for the first three months and quarterly thereafter for up to one year. Participants will be tested on a wide range of measures to evaluate physical function, vitality, cognition, cardiovascular disease, and sexual function.

Volunteering for a trial can really help advance research. Men interested in finding out more about participating in the study should call one of the following institutions:

- □ University of California, Los Angeles; 310-222-5297
- □ University of California, San Diego; 877-219-6610
- □ Boston University; 617-414-2968
- □ University of Pittsburgh; 800-872-3653
- □ Albert Einstein College of Medicine, Bronx, N.Y.; 718-405-8271
- □ Baylor College of Medicine, Houston, Texas; 713-798-8343
- □ University of Minnesota, Minneapolis; 612-625-4449
- □ Yale University, New Haven, Conn.; 203-737-5672
- □ University of Alabama at Birmingham; 205-934-2294
- □ *VA* Puget Sound Health Care System and University of Washington School of Medicine, Seattle; 206-768-5408
- □ Northwestern University, Evanston, Ill.; 877-300-3065
- □ University of Florida, Gainesville; 866-386-7730, 352-273-5919

Other Studies:

This is a list obtained from clinicaltrials.gov in summer of 2011 (visit the respective link to find out more about every study. This is a great way to not only have access to therapy, but also to have great monitoring and to serve for the better of humanity):

Title: Exogenous Testosterone plus Dutasteride for the Treatment of Castrate Metastatic Prostate Cancer
Recruitment: Recruiting
Conditions: Prostate Cancer|Castration-resistant, Metastatic
Interventions: Other: testosterone (AndroGel®) with the 5α-reductase inhibitor dutasteride
URL: http://ClinicalTrials.gov/show/NCT00853697

Title: Anabolic and Inflammatory Responses to Short-Term Testosterone Administration in Older Men
Recruitment: Recruiting
Conditions: Sarcopenia
Interventions: Drug: Testosterone injection|Drug: Testosterone gel
URL: http://ClinicalTrials.gov/show/NCT00957801

Title: Testosterone for Penile Rehab After Radical Prostatectomy
Recruitment: Recruiting
Conditions: Low Testosterone Levels|Erectile Dysfunction
Interventions: Drug: Testim® + Viagra®|Drug: Placebo Testim® + Viagra®
URL: http://ClinicalTrials.gov/show/NCT00848497

Title: Use of Nebido® to Assess Tolerability and Treatment Outcomes in Daily Clinical Practice
Recruitment: Recruiting
Conditions: Male|Hypogonadism
Interventions: Drug: Testosterone Undecanoate (Nebido, BAY86-5037)
URL: http://ClinicalTrials.gov/show/NCT00410306

Title: Pharmacokinetic and Comparative Bioavailability Study of Testosterone Absorption after Administration of Testosterone Gel 1.62% to the Upper Arms/Shoulders Using an Application Site Rotation or a Combination of Application Sites in Hypogonadal Males
Recruitment: Recruiting
Conditions: Hypogonadism
Interventions: Drug: Testosterone Gel 1.62%|Drug: Testosterone Gel 1.62%
URL: http://ClinicalTrials.gov/show/NCT01133548

Title: Effect of Testosterone on Endothelial Function and Microcirculation in Type 2 Diabetic Patients with Hypogonadism
Recruitment: Not yet recruiting
Conditions: Type 2 Diabetes|Hypogonadism
Interventions: Drug: Testosterone
URL: http://ClinicalTrials.gov/show/NCT01084369

Title: An Open-Label Study of Serum Testosterone Levels in Non-dosed Females After Secondary Exposure to Testosterone Gel 1.62% Applied to the Upper Arms and Shoulders and Use of a T-shirt Barrier

Recruitment: Recruiting
Conditions: Pharmacokinetics
Interventions: Drug: Testosterone Gel 1.62%
URL: http://ClinicalTrials.gov/show/NCT01130298

Title: Testosterone Replacement for Fatigue in Male Hypogonadic Advanced Cancer Patients
Recruitment: Recruiting
Conditions: Advanced Cancer
Interventions: Drug: Testosterone|Drug: Placebo
URL: http://ClinicalTrials.gov/show/NCT00965341

Title: Effect of Testosterone in Men with Erectile Dysfunction
Recruitment: Recruiting
Conditions: Erectile Dysfunction|Testosterone Deficiency|Diabetes
Interventions: Drug: Sildenafil citrate (open label)|Drug: Testosterone gel 1% (active or placebo)|Drug: Topical testosterone gel 1%
URL: http://ClinicalTrials.gov/show/NCT00512707

Title: Influence of Administration Route of Testosterone on Male Fertility
Recruitment: Not yet recruiting
Conditions: Hypogonadism
Interventions: Drug: MPP10, testosterone|Drug: Testosterone
URL: http://ClinicalTrials.gov/show/NCT00705796

Title: NASOBOL spray in Hypogonadal Men in Comparison to Testosterone Levels in Normal Healthy Male Volunteers
Recruitment: Recruiting
Conditions: Hypogonadism
Interventions: Drug: testosterone|Other: No treatment
URL: http://ClinicalTrials.gov/show/NCT00647868

Title: Effect of Testosterone Gel Replacement on Fat Mass in Males with Low Testosterone Levels and Diabetes
Recruitment: Not yet recruiting
Conditions: Hypogonadism|Diabetes
Interventions: Drug: Testosterone gel|Drug: placebo
URL: http://ClinicalTrials.gov/show/NCT00440440

Title: The Testosterone Trial
Recruitment: Recruiting

Conditions: Andropause
Interventions: Drug: AndroGel® (testosterone gel)
URL: http://ClinicalTrials.gov/show/NCT00799617

Title: Vaginal Testosterone Cream vs ESTRING for Vaginal Dryness or Decreased Libido in Early Stage Breast Cancer Patients
Recruitment: Recruiting
Conditions: Sexual Dysfunction, Physiological
Interventions: Drug: Testosterone Cream|Drug: Estring
URL: http://ClinicalTrials.gov/show/NCT00698035

Title: Effect of Testosterone Therapy in Men with Alzheimer's Disease and Low Testosterone
Recruitment: Recruiting
Conditions: Alzheimer's Disease|Hypogonadism
Interventions: Drug: AndroGel (Solvay Pharmaceuticals)
URL: http://ClinicalTrials.gov/show/NCT00392912

Title: 5-Alpha Reductase and Anabolic Effects of Testosterone
Recruitment: Recruiting
Conditions: Male Hypogonadism|Muscle Atrophy|Prostate Enlargement|Sarcopenia
Interventions: Drug: Testosterone Enanthate|Behavioral: Collection of 3-day food logs with counseling of subjects|Drug: Finasteride|Behavioral: Collection of 3-day food logs with counseling of subjects|Drug: Testosterone Enanthate|Drug: Finasteride|Behavioral: Collection of 3-day food logs with counseling of subjects
URL: http://ClinicalTrials.gov/show/NCT00475501

Title: Effects of Testosterone Replacement on Pain Sensitivity and Pain Perception
Recruitment: Recruiting
Study Results: No Results Available
Conditions: Pain|Hypogonadism
Interventions: Drug: Androgel (testosterone gel)|Other: Placebo
URL: http://ClinicalTrials.gov/show/NCT00351819

Title: Testosterone Gel Applied to Women with Pituitary Gland Problems
Recruitment: Recruiting
Conditions: Panhypopituitarism
Interventions: Drug: Transdermal Testosterone gel
URL: http://ClinicalTrials.gov/show/NCT00144391

Title: Testosterone Therapy in Men With Low Testosterone Levels and Metabolic Syndrome or Early Stages of Type 2 Diabetes
Recruitment: Recruiting
Conditions: Metabolic Syndrome
Interventions: Drug: Transdermal testosterone therapy|Drug: Placebo
URL: http://ClinicalTrials.gov/show/NCT00479609

Title: Effect of Testosterone Replacement on Insulin Resistance
Recruitment: Recruiting
Conditions: Metabolic Syndrome|Hypogonadism
Interventions: Radiation: Testosterone gel|Drug: Placebo for testosterone gel
URL: http://ClinicalTrials.gov/show/NCT00487734

Title: Effect of Androgel on Type 2 Diabetic Males with Hypogonadism
Recruitment: Recruiting
Conditions: Diabetes Mellitus Type 2
Interventions: Drug: Testosterone(AndroGel)
URL: http://ClinicalTrials.gov/show/NCT00350701

Title: TEAM: Testosterone Supplementation and Exercise in Elderly Men
Recruitment: Recruiting
Conditions: Healthy
Interventions: Drug: Testosterone Gel|Behavioral: Exercise - Progressive Resistance Training (PRT)|Drug: Placebo Gel
URL: http://ClinicalTrials.gov/show/NCT00112151

Title: Dose Titration Investigation of the Pharmacokinetics of Testosterone Transdermal Systems in Hypogonadal Men
Recruitment: Recruiting
Conditions: Hypogonadism
Interventions: Drug: Testerone Transdermal System
URL: http://ClinicalTrials.gov/show/NCT01104246

Title: Testosterone for Peripheral Vascular Disease
Recruitment: Recruiting
Conditions: Hypogonadism|Peripheral Vascular Disease|Type 2 Diabetes
Interventions: Drug: Testosterone|Drug: 0.9% saline
URL: http://ClinicalTrials.gov/show/NCT00504712

Title: **A Pilot Study of Parenteral Testosterone and Oral Etoposide as Therapy for Men with Castration Resistant Prostate Cancer**
Recruitment: Recruiting
Conditions: Prostate Cancer
Interventions: Drug: Testosterone|Drug: Etoposide
URL: http://ClinicalTrials.gov/show/NCT01084759

Title: **Efficacy and Tolerability of an Intra-Nasal Testosterone Product**
Recruitment: Recruiting
Conditions: Hypogonadism
Interventions: Drug: Nasobol® (Itra-nasal Testosterone)|Drug: Androderm® (Positive Control)
URL: http://ClinicalTrials.gov/show/NCT00975650

Title: **Testosterone Replacement in Men with Diabetes and Obesity**
Recruitment: Recruiting
Conditions: Hypogonadism
Interventions: Drug: testosterone|Drug: placebo
URL: http://ClinicalTrials.gov/show/NCT01127659

Title: **NEBIDO in Symptomatic Late Onset Hypogonadism (SLOH)**
Recruitment: Not yet recruiting
Conditions: Hypogonadism
Interventions: Drug: Testosterone Undeconate (Nebido, BAY86-5037)|Drug: Placebo
URL: http://ClinicalTrials.gov/show/NCT01092858

Title: **Baseline Sexual Function, Cognitive Function, Body Composition and Muscle Parameters and Pharmacokinetics of Transdermal Testosterone Gel in Women With Hypopituitarism**
Recruitment: Recruiting
Conditions: Panhypopituitarism
Interventions: Drug: Transdermal Testosterone Gel
URL: http://ClinicalTrials.gov/show/NCT00144404

Title: **Effect of Increasing Testosterone on Insulin Sensitivity in Men with the Metabolic Syndrome**
Recruitment: Recruiting
Conditions: Metabolic Syndrome
Interventions: Drug: Zoladex|Drug: AndroGel|Drug: Arimidex
URL: http://ClinicalTrials.gov/show/NCT00438321

Title: Testosterone Replacement in Men with Non-Metastatic Castrate Resistant Prostate Cancer
Recruitment: Recruiting
Conditions: Prostate Cancer
Interventions: Drug: AndroGel|Drug: placebo
URL: http://ClinicalTrials.gov/show/NCT00515112

Title: The Effect of IM Testosterone Undecanoate on Biochemical and Anthropometric Characteristics of Metabolic Syndrome in Hypogonadal Men
Recruitment: Recruiting
Conditions: Metabolic Syndrome|Hypogonadism
Interventions: Drug: Nebido (testosterone undecanoate)|Drug: Placebo
URL: http://ClinicalTrials.gov/show/NCT00696748

Title: The Therapy of Nebido as Mono or in Combination With PDE-5 Inhibitors in Hypogonadal Patients With Erectile Dysfunction
Recruitment: Recruiting
Conditions: Hypogonadism|Erectile Dysfunction
Interventions: Drug: Testosterone undecanoate
URL: http://ClinicalTrials.gov/show/NCT00421460

Title: Transdermal Testosterone Gel/Effect on Erection Quality as Measured by DIR
Recruitment: Recruiting
Conditions: Hypogonadism
Interventions: Drug: AndroGel (Transdermal Testosterone Gel)
URL: http://ClinicalTrials.gov/show/NCT00425568

Title: The Effect of 5-Alpha Reductase on Testosterone in Men
Recruitment: Recruiting
Conditions: Sex Disorders
Interventions: Drug: testosterone enanthate|Drug: duastride
URL: http://ClinicalTrials.gov/show/NCT00070733

Title: Treatment of Erectile Dysfunction in Hypogonadal Men with Testosterone Undecanoate
Recruitment: Recruiting
Conditions: Erectile Dysfunction|Hypogonadotrophic Males
Interventions: Drug: Testosterone Undecanoate and/or PDE-5
URL: http://ClinicalTrials.gov/show/NCT00555087

Title: Analgesic Efficacy of Testosterone Replacement in Hypogonadal Opioid-Treated Chronic Pain Patients: A Pilot Study.
Recruitment: Recruiting
Conditions: Pain|Hypogonadism
Interventions: Drug: Testosterone Gel
URL: http://ClinicalTrials.gov/show/NCT00398034

Title: Anabolic Therapies: New Hope for Treating Secondary Disabilities of SCI
Recruitment: Recruiting
Conditions: Hypogonadism|Spinal Cord Injury
Interventions: Drug: Testosterone Replacement Therapy Patch 5mg daily
URL: http://ClinicalTrials.gov/show/NCT00266864

Title: Does Testosterone Improve Function in Hypogonadal Older Men
Recruitment: Recruiting
Conditions: Hypogonadism
Interventions: Drug: Testosterone
URL: http://ClinicalTrials.gov/show/NCT00304213

Title: The Effect of Testosterone Replacement on Bone Mineral Density in Boys and Men with Anorexia Nervosa
Recruitment: Recruiting
Conditions: Bone Metabolism
Interventions: Drug: testosterone cypionate|Other: Bone monitoring
URL: http://ClinicalTrials.gov/show/NCT00853502

Title: Effects of Testosterone in Women with Depression
Recruitment: Recruiting
Conditions: Depression
Interventions: Drug: Testosterone
URL: http://ClinicalTrials.gov/show/NCT00676676

Title: Reandron in Diabetic Men With Low Testosterone Level
Recruitment: Recruiting
Conditions: Type 2 Diabetes|Hypogonadism
Interventions: Drug: Reandron 1000|Drug: placebo
URL: http://ClinicalTrials.gov/show/NCT00613782

Title: Outcomes of Mechanically Ventilated Patients With Low Serum Testosterone

Recruitment: Recruiting
Study Results: No Results Available
Conditions: Acute Respiratory Failure
Interventions:
URL: http://ClinicalTrials.gov/show/NCT00797433

Title: Testosterone Therapy **on Angina Threshold and Atheroma in Patients with Chronic Stable Angina**
Recruitment: Recruiting
Conditions: Angina Pectoris
Interventions: Drug: Nebido
URL: http://ClinicalTrials.gov/show/NCT00131183

Title: Hormone and Information Processing Study
Recruitment: Recruiting
Conditions: Mild Cognitive Impairment|Alzheimer's Disease
Interventions: Drug: testosterone gel|Drug: placebo gel
URL: http://ClinicalTrials.gov/show/NCT00539305

Title: Efficacy Study for Use of Dutasteride (Avodart) With Testosterone Replacement
Recruitment: Recruiting
Conditions: Hypogonadism
Interventions: Drug: dutasteride|Drug: placebo
URL: http://ClinicalTrials.gov/show/NCT00752869

Title: Testosterone Replacement in Middle-Aged Hypogonadal Men With Dysthymia: Parallel Group, Double Blind Randomized Trial
Recruitment: Recruiting
Conditions: Dysthymic Disorder
Interventions: Drug: Testoviron
URL: http://ClinicalTrials.gov/show/NCT00260390

Title: Decreased Testosterone Levels in Men Over 65
Recruitment: Recruiting
Conditions: Aging|Hypogonadism|Andropause
Interventions: Drug: Anastrozole|Drug: Testosterone Gel|Drug: Placebo tablet|Drug: Placebo gel|Dietary Supplement: Calcium Cardone 500mg with vitamin D 400 IU
URL: http://ClinicalTrials.gov/show/NCT00104572

Title: Testosterone Replacement Therapy in Advanced Chronic Kidney Disease
Recruitment: Recruiting
Study Results: No Results Available
Conditions: Kidney Failure|Kidney Diseases
Interventions: Drug: Testim (1% testosterone gel)
URL: http://ClinicalTrials.gov/show/NCT00645658

Title: The Cardiac Benefit of Testosterone Replacement in Men with Low Testosterone Levels With Coronary Artery Disease After Successful Intervention of the Blockage or Narrowed Heart Artery
Recruitment: Recruiting
Conditions: Coronary Artery Disease
Interventions: Drug: AndroGel 5 Grams
URL: http://ClinicalTrials.gov/show/NCT00413244

Title: Dose-Response of Gonadal Steroids and Bone Turnover in Men
Recruitment: Recruiting
Conditions: Healthy Volunteers
Interventions: Drug: testosterone|Drug: goserelin acetate|Drug: anastrazole
URL: http://ClinicalTrials.gov/show/NCT00114114

Title: Effect of Androgel on Atherogenesis, Inflammation, Cardiovascular Risk Factors and Adiposity in Type 2 Diabetic Males With Hypogonadotrophic Hypogonadism
Recruitment: Not yet recruiting
Conditions: Type 2 Diabetic Male with Hypogonadotrophic Hypogonadism.
Interventions: Drug: Androgel
URL: http://ClinicalTrials.gov/show/NCT00467987

Title: Hormonal Factors in the Treatment of Anorexia Nervosa
Recruitment: Recruiting
Conditions: Anorexia Nervosa|Eating Disorder|Anxiety|Depression
Interventions: Drug: Testosterone|Drug: Placebo
URL: http://ClinicalTrials.gov/show/NCT01121211

Title: Investigator Initiated Study of the Effects of Androgen Therapy on Carbohydrate and Lipid Metabolism In Elderly Men
Recruitment: Recruiting
Conditions: Aging|Obesity|Insulin Resistance|Hypogonadism

Interventions: Drug: Topical testosterone (Androgel) 10 g/day
URL: http://ClinicalTrials.gov/show/NCT00365794

Title: Phase II Randomized Study of Physiologic Testosterone Replacement in Premenopausal, HIV-Positive Women
Recruitment: Recruiting
Conditions: HIV Infections|Cachexia
Interventions: Drug: testosterone
URL: http://ClinicalTrials.gov/show/NCT00004400

Title: Amino Acid Supplement and/or Testosterone in Treating Cachexia in Patients With Advanced or Recurrent Cervical Cancer
Recruitment: Recruiting
Conditions: Cachexia|Cervical Cancer
Interventions: Dietary Supplement: leucine-enhanced essential amino acid dietary supplement|Drug: therapeutic testosterone|Other: placebo
URL: http://ClinicalTrials.gov/show/NCT00878995

Title: Deslorelin Combined With Low-Dose Add-Back Estradiol and Testosterone in Preventing Breast Cancer in Premenopausal Women Who Are at High Risk for This Disease
Recruitment: Recruiting
Conditions: brca1 Mutation Carrier|brca2 Mutation Carrier|Breast Cancer
Interventions: Biological: therapeutic estradiol|Drug: deslorelin|Drug: therapeutic testosterone
URL: http://ClinicalTrials.gov/show/NCT00080756

Title: Effect of High Testosterone on Sleep-associated Slowing of Follicular Luteinizing Hormone (LH) Frequency in Polycystic Ovary Syndrome
Recruitment: Recruiting
Conditions: Polycystic Ovary Syndrome
Interventions: Drug: Flutamide|Drug: Placebo
URL: http://ClinicalTrials.gov/show/NCT00930228

Title: Metabolic Effects of Androgenicity in Aging Men and Women
Recruitment: Recruiting
Conditions: Aging|Insulin Resistance
Interventions: Drug: Testosterone|Drug: Estrogen
URL: http://ClinicalTrials.gov/show/NCT00680797

Title: Sleep-wake Changes of Luteinizing Hormone Frequency in Pubertal Girls With and Without High Testosterone
Recruitment: Recruiting
Conditions: Hyperandrogenism
Interventions:
URL: http://ClinicalTrials.gov/show/NCT00930007

Title: Safety and Efficacy of LibiGel® for the Treatment of Hypoactive Sexual Desire Disorder in Surgically Menopausal Women
Recruitment: Recruiting
Conditions: Hypoactive Sexual Desire Disorder
Interventions: Drug: testosterone gel|Drug: placebo gel
URL: http://ClinicalTrials.gov/show/NCT00613002

Title: Safety and Efficacy of LibiGel® for Treatment of Hypoactive Sexual Desire Disorder in Postmenopausal Women
Recruitment: Recruiting
Conditions: Hypoactive Sexual Desire Disorder
Interventions: Drug: testosterone gel|Drug: placebo gel
URL: http://ClinicalTrials.gov/show/NCT00612742

Title: Sexual Dysfunction and Hypotestosteronemia In Patients With Obstructive Sleep Apnea Syndrome And Its Effects With CPAP Therapy
Recruitment: Recruiting
Conditions: Obstructive Sleep Apnea Syndrome (OSAS)|Sleep Apnea|Hypotestosteronemia
Interventions:
URL: http://ClinicalTrials.gov/show/NCT00832065

Title: Surveillance Study of Women Taking Intrinsa®
Recruitment: Recruiting
Study Results: No Results Available
Conditions: Ovariectomy|Hysterectomy|Hypoactive Sexual Desire Disorder
Interventions:
URL: http://ClinicalTrials.gov/show/NCT00551785

Title: Safety and Efficacy of LibiGel® for Treatment of Hypoactive Sexual Desire Disorder in Surgically Menopausal Women
Recruitment: Recruiting
Conditions: Hypoactive Sexual Desire Disorder

Interventions: Drug: testosterone gel|Drug: placebo gel
URL: http://ClinicalTrials.gov/show/NCT00657501

Interventions: Procedure: Stable Isotope Infusion Study|Procedure: Collection of blood and tissues|Procedure: Radiology testing: DEXA, K+ counter, ultrasound, MRI|Drug: Humatrope|Drug: Ketoconazole|Drug: Oxandrolone|Drug: Propranolol|Drug: Oxandrolone and propranolol combined|Drug: Humatrope and propranolol combined|Drug: Placebo|Behavioral: Exercise--Hospital supervised intensive exercise program|Behavioral: Home exercise program
URL: http://ClinicalTrials.gov/show/NCT00675714

Title: Registry of Hypogonadism in Men
Recruitment: Recruiting
Conditions: Male Hypogonadism|Androgen Deficiency|Testosterone Deficiency
Interventions: Other: Standard of Care
URL: http://ClinicalTrials.gov/show/NCT00858650

Title: Sex Steroids, Sleep, and Metabolic Dysfunction in Women
Recruitment: Recruiting
Study Results: No Results Available
Conditions: Polycystic Ovary Syndrome|Obstructive Sleep Apnea|Obesity
Interventions: Drug: Progesterone|Drug: testosterone|Drug: glucocorticoid|Device: continuous positive airway pressure
URL: http://ClinicalTrials.gov/show/NCT00805207

Title: Studying the Effects of 7 Days of Gonadotropin Releasing Hormone (GnRH) Treatment in Men with Hypogonadism
Recruitment: Recruiting
Conditions: Kallmann Syndrome|Idiopathic Hypogonadotropic Hypogonadism
Interventions: Drug: gonadotropin releasing hormone (GnRH)
URL: http://ClinicalTrials.gov/show/NCT00493961

Title: Follicle Stimulating Hormone (FSH) to Improve Testicular Development in Men with Hypogonadism
Recruitment: Recruiting
Conditions: Hypogonadism|Kallmann Syndrome
Interventions: Procedure: Testicular biopsy|Drug: gonadotropin releasing hormone (GnRH)|Drug: follicle stimulating hormone (FSH)
URL: http://ClinicalTrials.gov/show/NCT00064987

Title: Prevalence of Hypogonadism in Male Cancer Patients
Recruitment: Recruiting
Conditions: Cancer|Hypogonadism
Interventions:
URL: http://ClinicalTrials.gov/show/NCT00472940

Index

A

acne 7, 9, 22, 43, 57, 69, 71, 92, 93, 140, 152
Adderall 112, 113, 114
adrenal function 108
alcohol 6, 12, 14, 22, 34, 35, 36, 43, 52, 55, 83, 98, 100, 110, 151
anabolic steroids 2, 19, 58, 69, 89, 90, 94, 96, 132, 133, 134, 144, 145, 146, 148
anastrazole 59, 87, 98, 163, 176
Andriol 24, 140
Androderm 45, 46
AndroGel 170, 171, 172, 173, 176
Arimidex 54, 59, 89, 154, 163, 164, 172
Aveed 28, 32, 63
Azoospermia 89

B

benign prostatic hyperplasia ix, 75, 133, 139
blood pressure 24, 28, 76, 77, 78, 80, 81, 82, 87, 88, 89, 98, 100, 101, 102, 103, 109, 110, 117, 121, 125, 150
blood pressure medications 82
BPH ix, 75, 76, 77, 78, 133, 139

C

Cachexia 177
Cancer 67, 73, 75, 76, 84, 167, 169, 170, 172, 173, 177, 180
cardiovascular iii, 2, 26, 28, 65, 66, 82, 86, 87, 88, 89, 100, 110, 113, 120, 121, 126, 133, 134, 136, 146, 167
Caverjet 105
Cholesterol xi, 85, 108
Cialis 65, 70, 99, 102, 104, 105, 119
Clomid 154
clomiphene citrate 59, 60, 96, 146, 147, 148
compounded gels 26
compounding pharmacies iii, 20, 25, 30, 31, 43, 44, 47, 49, 50, 51, 52, 57, 58, 60, 68, 94, 103, 105, 160, 161, 162, 163, 164
coronary artery disease 85, 86

CPAP 110, 111, 114, 178

D

DEA ix, 19, 60, 112
depo testosterone 96, 141
DEXA 120, 179
DHEA ix, 12, 16, 109, 110, 115
DHT ix, 7, 28, 29, 41, 43, 44, 45, 46, 48, 53, 54, 58, 63, 71, 76, 77, 83, 92, 93, 139, 143
Drug Enforcement Agency ix, 19, 60

E

ejaculate 93, 139
erectile dysfunction 10, 60, 76, 82, 98, 100, 105, 106, 107, 116, 117, 139
estradiol 7, 28, 53, 54, 56, 58, 59, 60, 70, 72, 76, 82, 83, 84, 87, 88, 89, 91, 98, 110, 140, 143, 164, 177
estrogen ix, 7, 12, 16, 38, 45, 48, 54, 56, 59, 72, 83, 84, 87, 88, 96, 109, 110, 130, 139, 140, 147, 166
exercise iii, viii, 1, 22, 48, 80, 82, 88, 89, 114, 120, 121, 125, 126, 127, 128, 129, 130, 134, 155, 179

F

fatigue vii, 6, 67, 79, 81, 108, 109, 110, 112, 113, 114, 121, 129, 137
fertility 54, 59, 90, 118, 144, 145
finasteride 76, 77, 84, 93, 139, 154
Flomax 76, 77
Fortesta 44, 63
free testosterone 7, 8, 12, 13, 14, 15, 17, 26, 56, 85, 142, 143
FSH ix, 5, 6, 11, 12, 13, 59, 90, 95, 144, 180

G

ginseng 115, 116, 119
growth hormone ix, 50, 68, 81, 116, 119, 121
guidelines 53, 158, 159
gym 126, 128
gynecomastia 7, 57, 68, 72, 83, 84, 87, 110, 139, 146, 164

H

hair loss 7, 9, 22, 43, 92, 93, 139

HCG ix, xiii, 50, 51, 52, 53, 54, 55, 56, 57, 58, 59, 60, 90, 93, 94, 96, 97, 98, 99, 146, 147, 163, 164, 166

hematocrit 28, 69, 71, 72, 78, 79, 80, 87, 88, 89, 136, 137, 138, 139, 143

HIV iii, vii, viii, 1, 2, 33, 66, 67, 68, 71, 79, 80, 83, 84, 85, 91, 92, 93, 96, 101, 102, 114, 132, 165, 177

HPGA ix, xi, 5, 6, 12, 21, 58, 59, 60, 67, 69, 94, 95, 96, 97, 144, 145, 166

HPTA ix, 97, 132, 138, 144, 145, 147, 148

human chorionic gonadotropin ix, 98, 147

hypogonadism iii, 2, 3, 6, 9, 10, 11, 12, 13, 19, 55, 58, 59, 60, 63, 69, 81, 96, 108, 132, 134, 135, 138, 140, 142, 145, 146, 147, 148, 156, 164

hypothalamic-pituitary-gonadal axis ix, 5

I

immune system 1, 118

injection 21, 25, 26, 27, 28, 29, 31, 32, 33, 35, 36, 37, 38, 51, 52, 53, 54, 56, 57, 58, 63, 68, 71, 94, 95, 104, 105, 137, 141, 142, 168

Internet Discussion Groups 155

K

ketoconazole 93, 102

L

Levitra 65, 70, 99, 104, 105

LH ix, 5, 6, 11, 12, 13, 50, 59, 60, 69, 90, 95, 98, 144, 147, 148, 177

LibiGel 64, 65

liver 1, 6, 12, 21, 24, 29, 30, 48, 49, 67, 68, 69, 81, 92, 99, 100, 101, 102, 113, 114, 117, 119, 133, 140, 143

low sperm count 89, 95

M

maca 118

marijuana 84

mental 9, 10, 91, 113

Michael Scally iv, xi, 60, 79, 96, 131, 148

mixed hypogonadism 6

mood 2, 5, 7, 9, 10, 33, 60, 71, 85, 91, 92, 121, 125

muscle 4, 5, 20, 30, 36, 37, 66, 67, 68, 76, 78, 85, 87, 89, 94, 96, 97, 100, 103, 111, 115, 120, 122, 125, 126, 127, 128, 129, 130, 132,

133, 139, 143, 146, 153
muscular 128
Muse 103

N

nandrolone 67, 68, 80, 81, 85
Nebido 32, 33, 63, 168, 172, 173, 175
nutrition iii, viii, 1, 129, 155

O

Omega 3 121, 124, 129
overtraining 128, 129
oxandrolone 67, 68, 85

P

patient assistance programs iii, 3, 20
pellets 23, 38, 46, 47, 48, 78
penile restriction rings 105
penis 4, 42, 75, 103, 104, 105, 116, 117
phlebotomy 71, 79, 80, 87, 88, 138, 166
polycythemia 68, 78, 79, 80, 81, 87, 136, 137, 138, 139, 146, 166
primary hypogonadism 12, 55, 60
prolactin 12, 13
Proscar 76, 108, 139
prostate 1, 61, 67, 73, 74, 75, 76, 77, 78, 84, 93, 101, 102, 108, 117, 133,
            135, 136, 139, 143, 150
prostatic specific antigen ix, 22, 69, 71, 72, 135
prostatitis 75
PSA ix, 22, 69, 71, 72, 74, 75, 135, 136, 143, 150

R

resistance exercise 126
resources 164, 165
Ritalin 112

S

SARM 143
saw palmetto 77, 119
secondary hypogonadism 59, 147, 164

selective androgen receptor modulators ix, 66, 143
Serostim 68
sex hormone binding globulin ix, 8, 88
sexual dysfunction 2, 64, 66, 70, 81, 82, 98, 107, 108
SHBG ix, 8, 12, 13, 14, 15, 142, 143
Shippen 38, 54, 55, 56
Sleep apnea 108, 110, 111
Spanish vi, 68
stimulants 112, 113, 121
Striant 49, 140
Sustanon 30, 31, 33, 96
syringes 33, 34, 44, 51, 52, 54, 105

T

tamoxifen 54, 58, 60, 83, 96, 146, 147, 148, 164
testicular atrophy 50, 57, 58, 94, 164, 166
Testim 29, 38, 41, 42, 43, 44, 63, 133, 140, 141, 155, 156, 176
Testoderm 45, 46
Testopel 46, 47, 48
testosterone cypionate 1, 25, 27, 30, 31, 57, 68, 96, 141, 144, 174
testosterone enanthate 25, 28, 30, 33, 38, 53, 137, 141, 173
testosterone undecanoate 23, 24, 81, 117, 140, 173
TestosteroneWisdom.com vi, 3, 37, 43, 94, 155, 163
thyroid 98, 108, 114, 132, 165
Total testosterone 8, 21
Tribulus 118, 119
Trimix 103, 104, 105
TSH 108

V

Viagra 65, 70, 99, 101, 104, 105, 106, 116, 117, 118, 119

W

wasting syndrome vii, 1, 67, 68, 96, 138
water retention 7, 9, 54, 57, 68, 82, 83, 110
whey protein 124, 129
women iv, 3, 12, 13, 17, 26, 44, 47, 50, 59, 64, 65, 66, 68, 72, 82, 84, 90, 109, 110, 118, 120, 125, 130, 134

Y

yohimbine 103, 117

Z

zinc 92, 93, 118

CPSIA information can be obtained at www.ICGtesting.com
Printed in the USA
LVOW012315130911

246096LV00002B/2/P

9 780966 223125